The Lies
Beneath
The Mask

The Lies Beneath The Mask

written by
Linda Nucci

RoseDog ✦ Books
PITTSBURGH, PENNSYLVANIA 15222

ISBN # 0-8059-9484-X
Printed in the United States of America

First Printing

For information or to order additional books, please write:
RoseDog Books
701 Smithfield St.
Pittsburgh, PA 15222
U.S.A.
1-800-834-1803
Or visit our web site and
on-line bookstore at www.rosedogbookstore.com

PREFACE

Bob is an Executive Officer of a very large corporation. He has an extensive education and has worked very hard to earn the position he now holds with this company. He is a very intelligent and responsible person, and is respected by all that know him.

One afternoon Bob was driving to a very important meeting. His previous meeting had taken an hour longer than expected, and he was now behind on his schedule. He was approaching a stop sign at the intersection of a road that he had frequently passed through, and he recalled that each time he had previously stopped there he had never seen any other vehicles in the area. In his effort to be prompt he decides that this time he won't bother stopping for the stop sign. As he drives past the stop sign there is suddenly another vehicle right in the middle of the intersection. It's too late and he can't stop his car. He hits the other vehicle, and although he doesn't sustain any serious injuries, the other driver is killed. One wrong decision has just taken another man's life.

Bob is absolutely shattered, but no matter how badly he feels, or how responsible he has been in the past, his disregard for the stop sign has just made him a murderer. He begins to panic and he thinks about everything he will lose as a result of his negligence. There is nothing he can do to restore the other man's life, but maybe he can save his own life and career from being destroyed.

Bob then steps further out of character and he decides to lie about what happened. He told the police that after he had stopped for the stop sign he proceeded to drive across the intersection but the other driver must have ignored his stop sign. He then stated that the other vehicle was suddenly in front of him, and although he tried, it was too late for him to stop.

An investigation was conducted. The length of the skid marks in the road, and the speed and point of impact on the other vehicle were facts that proved that Bob was lying. Bob went to jail for vehicular manslaughter.

The stop sign wasn't just a warning for Bob to adhere to if he had chosen. It was placed at that intersection for a good reason, as all stop signs are. The need to stop for it was the law. Bob had broken that law, and his failure to uphold the responsibility that came with his license to drive had caused harm to another person. Bob will pay for his mistake for the rest of his life.

In a hospital operating room a man has just undergone abdominal surgery. The man's surgery had taken an hour longer than was expected. Another surgery is scheduled to take place in the same operating room, and now the anesthesiologist is an hour behind on his schedule. To recover some lost time he has the patient quickly moved from the operating room table to a hospital bed in preparation for his transfer to the recovery room. Although untimely for the patient's condition, the anesthesiologist decides to remove the patient's breathing tube. The patient's ability to breathe on his own appears to be stable. To further expedite the patient's transfer, and contrary to the protocols in place to insure a patient's safety, the anesthesiologist decides he won't waste time reconnecting the patient to the oxygen or to any monitors.

Although aware that allowing the operating room to be cleaned, or a "Room turnover" as it's called, with the patient still present in the room is against hospital protocol, the anesthesiologist recalls having done this on numerous other occasions, and has never encountered any complications. He knows that if he is completely prepared for the next surgery, when he does deliver the patient to the recovery room, his work with this patient will be completed, and this will allow him to quickly move on to his next case. He is confident the patient will be fine, and he leaves him on the hospital bed in front of the doors he will exit with him when his work is completed.

A room turnover is initiated. Technicians arrive and start to clean the used equipment and restock the supplies. The medical staff is busy removing the instruments to be sterilized and completing their documentation in the patient's medical chart.

The anesthesiologist begins preparing the medications he will need to start the next surgery. His back is to the patient, and after approximately fifteen minutes he suddenly hears someone shout; "Hey, is there something wrong here? Is this suppose to be this way?" Everyone in the room turns to look, and can see that the patient's color is now dark blue. The medical staff quickly responds to the patient knowing that their failure to properly monitor him has now caused him to suffer a great deal of harm.

The anesthesiologist immediately begins taking all the necessary steps to reinsert a breathing tube into the patient. He knows that to become dark blue the patient had been deprived of oxygen for a very long time. He also knew that to be dark blue meant that the patient had already suffered severe anoxic brain damage.

After several minutes he had successfully reinserted another breathing tube into the patient's airway, and the monitors were then reconnected to the patient. The monitors immediately signaled that the patient's heart was beginning to dysfunction from the duration of time he had been deprived of oxygen. The anesthesiologist, still busy trying to manage the patient's airway, now realized that he needed help to save the patient's failing heart. He knows that if he calls a code to obtain that help many doctors would respond. The patient's condition and the sequence of events that had occurred could expose his negligence. He does not call for help.

Unexpectedly another anesthesiologist just happens by the operating room, and quickly responds to the patient's cardiac needs. He stabilizes the patient, but is unaware of the events prior to his entering the room. He leaves believing the patient is now okay. The patient, although physically stable, is severely brain damaged, and will remain so for the rest of his life.

The anesthesiologist begins to panic, and as badly as he now feels, he knows there is nothing he can do to reverse the damage that has occurred to the patient's brain. He could however save his own life and career from being destroyed, and he decides he will lie and place the blame of the brain damage on the patient's heart.

When the surgeon returned to the operating room, the anesthesiologist told him that the minute he had removed the patient's breathing tube he realized that the patient was in distress. He further stated that he had immediately replaced the breathing tube and secured the patient's airway, leaving the surgeon with very little concern that the patient had suffered any harm. The patient was then transferred to the recovery room.

Several hours later the surgeon was becoming increasingly concerned because the patient was not awake and as responsive as he should be. He called for a neurologist to determine if something was wrong with the patient.

After a physical examination and reviewing the results of the tests he had performed, the neurologist concludes that the patient has suffered a severe and irreversible brain damage due to a prolonged period of time with a lack of oxygen. He finds no evidence that the patient's heart had contributed to his present condition.

A Cardiologist is then called to examine the patient's heart. After a physical examination and reviewing the results of the tests he had performed, the cardiologist concludes that the patient's heart had not contributed in any way to the damage of his brain. He does however conclude that a long period of time with a lack of oxygen had definitely caused his heart to dysfunction.

The type and severity of damage to the patient's brain, the test results, and the diagnosis of the two specialists were proof that the anesthesiologist was lying.

Unlike Bob, the anesthesiologist was not held responsible, and suffered no consequences for his negligence that had destroyed this man's life.

What is the difference between Bob and the anesthesiologist? Absolutely nothing! They were both intelligent, successful, and very respected men. Both of them had unintentionally but carelessly taken another man's life.

But a driver's license comes with laws that the State mandates must be obeyed, and to take a life by not adhering to the law is considered murder. The doctor's license to practice medicine does not come with any laws, and the State does not consider medical negligence murder.

The State holds the responsibility of a driver's license to higher standards than a license to practice medicine and the Federal Government fails to recognize the obvious as to why medical errors are on the rise. I find this very disturbing, and if you don't then maybe the following will.

WASHINGTON (CNN) A federal advisory panel reported that more people die each year in the United States from medical errors than from highway accidents, breast cancer, or AIDS. The report from the National Academy of Sciences' Institute of Medicine cited studies showing between 44,000 and 98,000 people die each year because of mistakes by medical professionals. "That's probable an underestimate for two reasons," noted Dr. Donald Berwick of the Institute of Medicine. "One is, there are many different kinds of errors we never learn about - - even in retrospective studies - - because they are never written down. And second, these studies did not include other areas of care, like home care, nursing homes, and ambulatory care centers," Berwick said.

"The groundbreaking report urged Congress to create a National Center for Patient Safety within the Department of Health and Human Services to set goals for avoiding medical mistakes, track progress in meeting them and to fund research on better ways to prevent such errors."

Congress responds by introducing a bill that would put a cap on compensatory damages awarded to plaintiffs' in medical malpractice lawsuits. This bill further supports the negligence of doctors, and completely ignores the needs of the patients they have harmed. They continue to frown on the lawsuits that are brought against doctors, yet they fail to hold them accountable for their actions, and to provide the public with any form of assurance to protect their lives. They assume that all medical professionals are honest, and continue to hold them above any laws, leaving those that have been harmed no choice but to seek justice through a private lawsuit.

Now, adding insult to injury, they put their efforts into controlling the amount awarded in these lawsuits, instead of implementing some control of the doctors. Through their ignorance they have created their own monsters, and the public, as usual, is left to pay for that ignorance.

The number of medical errors will continue to rise until Congress addresses the need to provide laws under which medical professionals practice, and mandate consequences if these laws are broken. It's time to stop the medical community from policing itself, and take measures that give medical professionals a greater motive to adhere to stop signs.

The field of medicine is very complex and many are the times that unfortunate circumstances are beyond any doctor or nurse's control. Outside of these circumstances there are no acceptable excuses for compromising a patient's life. Mistakes can easily be made, but over the years as mistakes have been made medical facilities have created protocols to prevent careless mistakes from being repeated. Some mistakes can be small and some can be big, but make no mistake that both can be deadly. The list of potential errors are many, and to ignore the protocols that prevent these errors is a profound disregard for a patient's life, and is without question negligence.

Following protocols is the only assurance that medicine offers for a patient to receive safe care regardless how busy a doctor or a nurse is. Each time a protocol is broken a patient is knowingly put at a higher risk to be harmed. Ignoring a protocol is no different than ignoring a stop sign.

While adherence to protocols will not prevent all medical errors, as stop signs do not prevent all accidents, repeatedly preventable errors in medical facilities are traced back to an ignored protocol. The Department of Health, although aware of this, turns a blind eye to the conduct of the medical professionals who have failed to adhere, even when knowing that this conduct has caused a patient to be harmed. The DOH operates within the guidelines of the New York State Public Health Law. This law requires that a doctor only needs to meet minimal standards to practice medicine, and is only required to provide minimal care to their patients. They do not consider doctors' failure to adhere to the protocols of the facility in which they practice medicine to be negligence, because protocols are merely guidelines, and are not enforceable laws. This leaves the question of who protects the public? The answer is a frightening "No one."

The Government's failure to protect the public has left the threat of a lawsuit the only option a patient has to ensure that a doctor renders good care. Although the vast majority of doctors do practice above minimal standards and do adhere to protocols, there are far too many that don't. Although the vast majority of nurses provide safe patient care, and do adhere to protocols, there are far too many that don't. The later of these two serve as catalysts for errors, and without the threat of serious consequences this will never change. Their negligence will continue to contaminate the medical profession.

Until the Federal Government takes measures that force the State to raise the standards of practicing medicine, and to change protocols into laws that do come with consequences if broken, needless medical errors will continue to rise. For too long medical organizations have been allowed to hide their mistakes behind their own flexible rules. For too long the careless taking of another's life has been excused by a title.

INTRODUCTION

As the nurse wheeled Joe into the operating room, he looked back, stretched his arm out to me and said, "Lin, I'm scared, I'm really scared." I replied, "I know Joe, I love you, and I'll be right here for you when you come out." I tried not to let him see the tears that were beginning to fill my eyes, but the nurse did, and she looked at me and said "Don't worry, we'll take good care of him." Feeling a lump in my throat, I mouthed "Thank you."

I didn't know that would be the last time I would tell my husband of 27 years that I loved him and he would be able to understand me. Nowhere in my deepest concerns for his well being did I ever imagine that after the surgery they would return him to me severely and irreversibly brain damaged, but that's what they did. That was nine years ago, and to this day Joe continues to live in a state of vegetation.

I relive the memory of that day over and over, and the pain and anger grow more intense with time. My heart aches every day as I think of him lying in the operating room, desperate for just one breath, a breath that would have saved his life, and left him the normal functioning person he was when he went into that operating room. I can't imagine the fear and the pain of the suffocation he experienced. He was in a room with doctors and nurses who easily should have been able to help him had they been paying attention to him. But they were not, nor was he on any monitors, and no one noticed he wasn't breathing until he turned dark blue. Dark blue meant that his heart could no longer function due to lack of oxygen. Dark blue meant he had already suffered too much damage for any intervention to be effective. Dark blue meant he was deprived of oxygen for a very long time without being noticed.

CHAPTER 1

It was July of 1994. My husband Joe and our sons Joe Jr. and Nick had taken a short trip to Petersburg Virginia to view Joe Sr.'s display in the Softball Hall of Fame. Joe had been inducted for his accomplishments as a coach in the USSA Softball Organization. He was not only instrumental in the development of the organization on a national level, but he was the only coach to have delivered a "Softball World Championship" title to Rochester. He was very respected in the organization, as well as in the community, and we were all very proud of him. Our sons were anxious to see his display, as they too were now involved in playing softball, and were hearing many stories about their dad from men who had played ball for him. He had been quite the colorful coach.

Many things were planned for the months ahead. Joe Jr. was getting married in August, and Nick was going to return to college at the University of Rochester in September. Joe and I would be celebrating our 27th wedding anniversary on August 26th. We had a long awaited vacation planned in November for just the two of us. We would fly to Virginia so he and I could see his display together, and then fly on to Vegas to meet some friends. With our children now grown and leaving home, when we returned, we planned to start looking for a home to purchase that would better suit just the two of us.

We had accomplished raising a beautiful family, and our marriage had survived all of the obstacles that life had to offer us over the years.

We had now reached a place in our lives that all couples look forward to from the first day of their marriage. We were about to begin a new phase of togetherness. We both felt especially fortunate because we were still young; Joe was 47 and I 45. We would have many years ahead of us to enjoy watching our children and grandchildren grow, and could still remain an active part of their lives.

Now was the perfect time for Joe and our sons to make the trip. They left on Friday and were planning to return home on Monday. All did not go as planned, and they returned home on Sunday. Joe Sr. had eaten spicy chicken wings on Saturday night, and was now experiencing severe abdominal cramps. Two years prior Joe had been diagnosed with diverticulosis, a common condition in which pouches form in the intestine, and may easily become inflamed, allowing an infection to develop. When an infection settles in the pouches can become large and obstruct the intestine causing great discomfort. The condition is then called diverticulitis. A bland diet and taking fiber is the normal course of action to keep diverticulitis at bay.

For the past two years Joe had done a very good job maintaining a proper diet and was keeping good control of the diverticulosis. The bland diet had also helped him to lose weight. He had already lost fifty pounds, and was now walking daily along with his diet in an effort to lose even more. He still weighed about two hundred pounds, but I was really impressed with his accomplishments in taking off the weight. Joe had been very conscious of his diet, and now the one time he had cheated he was paying very dearly for it.

As the week passed, Joe's abdominal discomfort had not only persisted, but had become much worse. Nothing he did had given him any relief, and the signs were obvious that pouches had formed and were causing some obstruction in his intestine. I urged him to call our doctor, but he felt very strongly that it would resolve if he just took some fiber and ate the proper foods. This had always worked in the past, but it was not working this time. On Saturday morning when I awoke at 4:30 am for work, I found Joe on the sofa holding his stomach, and groaning with pain. Now I was convinced he had an obstruction, and I insisted he go to the emergency department. He agreed, and I took him to Rochester General Hospital.

When we arrived at the hospital, I informed the emergency room doctor of Joe's condition and the symptoms he had experienced through the prior week. He drew some blood and sent it to the lab to be processed, and then he proceeded with this physical examination of Joe. He knew I was a nurse, and when the lab results came back he reviewed them with me. None of the results were outside of normal parameters. He did however, based on his physical examination, Joe's symptoms, and the history over the past week, determine that an obstruction could be very possible. He admitted Joe to the hospital so that he could receive a course of conservative medical intervention. This would entail resting the bowel by not eating, antibiotics for the suspected infection, stool softeners, and analgesics to relieve the pain. If this intervention worked, Joe would be relieved and discharged in a couple of days.

Our family doctor, Avie Grunspan, was on vacation at the time of Joe's admission, and Dr. Michael Myers was seeing his patients until he returned. Dr. Myers came to see Joe that evening and agreed with the plan of care that was in place. We also discussed the possible need for surgery if all did not go as planned.

Over the next couple of days Joe's pain was not relieved, and on Monday he was scheduled for further tests. On Tuesday a GI specialist performed what is called a flexible sigmoidoscopy on Joe. This test entailed running a soft probe with a camera on the end of it through the colon to obtain an internal view. At the completion of the sigmoidoscopy the specialist informed us that he did in fact find some pouches and irritation in the intestine, but he felt that with a few medication changes a conservative course of action would still be effective and surgery would not be needed at this time. They initiated the change of medications, and Joe was scheduled for discharge on Wednesday. I was very reluctant to take Joe home because of the severity of pain that continued to persist, but I could only rely on the test results and hope that the specialist was correct in his diagnosis.

I had been with Joe every day since his admission to the hospital, and I needed to return to work on Wednesday. I made arrangements to pick him up from the hospital and take him home Wednesday after work. On Wednesday morning, while at work, I received a frantic call from Joe. He told me that a surgeon had now informed him that they needed to perform surgery as soon as possible. I told Joe to have the surgeon meet me in his room at 6pm that evening.

I arrived in Joe's room at approximately 5:30 pm, and the surgeon arrived shortly thereafter. The surgeon was Dr. Peter Wojdylo. I knew Dr. Wojdylo, and had once been a patient of his myself. I asked him what had taken place to cause such a sudden change in Joe's condition that now required surgery. Dr. Wojdylo explained that late Tuesday night Joe's pain had become even more severe than it had been, and that his abdomen was now even more distended. An X-ray Tuesday night found the narrowing in his colon had now caused a complete obstruction that even air could not pass through. The obstruction was causing an increased pressure in the colon, which was the cause of the further distention and the increased pain. By now Joe's abdomen had become extremely large and very hard. Surgery to remove the damaged segment of bowel was the only option for relief, and it had to be done as soon as possible to prevent any further damage.

Joe had been suffering for ten long days, and I couldn't stand seeing him in such relentless pain any longer. I also knew that Joe was afraid to have surgery, and I didn't want him to stress about it any longer than was necessary. I asked Dr. Wojdylo to perform the surgery that night. He stated that there was no further risk to Joe if he waited until morning, and that he would rather perform the surgery with a fresh and rested staff. Surgery was then scheduled for morning. I stayed with Joe until late that night. I helped him to bathe, and made small talk to keep his mind off of the pending surgery.

Our son's wedding was scheduled for August 20th, and Joe was worried he would not be able to attend. He made me promise I would get him there even if it had to be in a wheelchair. I told him I would make whatever arrangements had to be made, but I would not let him miss it. I stayed with him until he fell asleep, and then I went home so I could rest and be back early in the morning to be with him before he went into the operating room. When I got home I informed our family that he was scheduled for surgery in the morning.

CHAPTER II

On Thursday, August 11th, I arrived at the hospital just after 7:30 am. Joe was awake and waiting for me. Again he started talking about missing the wedding. Again, I assured him that I wouldn't let that happen. I was happy that his focus was on something other than the operation, so I encouraged the conversation. Finally, just before 9:00 am, the nurse came in to give him a sedative. We then went to what is called the " Holding Tank" a room outside of the operating room, where people who are having surgery are taken just before going in.

When we arrived in the Holding Tank, a man approached us wearing hospital scrubs and a cap. He said, "Hi, I'm Dr. Proper, the anesthesiologist that will be taking care of Joe during his surgery this morning." He barely got the words out of this mouth when he was called over to the window at the nurse's station. Dr. Proper never came back to us, and then a nurse came out of the operating room to take Joe back in. As she was wheeling the gurney away from me, the fear of the surgery must have suddenly kicked into Joe's thoughts. He stretched his arm out to me and said, "Lin, I'm scared, I'm really scared." I felt sick seeing him so afraid and so helpless, but I knew if he saw how I was feeling it would only make him feel worse. The nurse stopped the gurney and I went to Joe and took his hand. I said "I know Joe, I love you and I'll be right here for you when you come out." I kissed him and stepped back so he couldn't see me, as I could now feel my eyes beginning to fill with tears. The nurse looked at me and said, "Don't worry, we'll take good care of him." She then took Joe into the operating room, and I went to the lobby where I had been told to wait. The surgeon would meet me there when the surgery over. Dr. Wojdylo had informed me that the surgery would take anywhere from two to four hours, depending on how much damage he found after he had opened Joe's abdomen.

When I got to the lobby, our son Nick, our daughter Daneane, Joe's father Nick, and his cousin, Joe, were there to meet me. I was happy to see them, as I really needed the support, as well as some distraction from my concerns, and the thoughts of Joe's fear. We talked the time away for a while, but once three hours had passed I began feeling very anxious. It was now going into the fourth hour, and I couldn't stop thinking about what Dr. Wojdylo might have found that was taking so long. I started watching the clock and praying.

Finally, at 2:05 p.m., I saw Dr. Wojdylo coming down the hall. He was wearing his suit, but more importantly he was wearing a smile. Dr. Wojdylo proceeded to tell me that the surgery had gone well. He did however say that a larger portion of Joe's intestine had been affected than he had originally thought. He said the pressure from the obstruction had caused damage in another area, which he was able to repair. He also told me that they had a room ready for Joe on the fourth floor, but he wanted to send him to the Surgical Intensive Care Unit (SICU) first. He felt that Joe would benefit from the closer observation and would be able to receive extra pain medications in the SICU as opposed to the floor unit. Either way, he said I could see him in about one hour. I thanked him, as did everyone with me.

Feeling relief from the good news, the air lightened. We stood in the lobby and made small talk for a short while. Joe's dad and cousin decided to leave and return later to see Joe after he had awoken. Our son Nick had to leave for work at 2:30 p.m., and asked me to tell his dad he would be back to see him after work. Daneane and I stayed to be with Joe.

It was now 2:25 p.m., and we were all standing in the lobby saying our good-byes when we saw Dr. Wojdylo coming back down the hall. He then informed me that when the attempt was made to extubate Joe (remove his breathing tube), "He didn't do so well", but that he had been immediately reintubated, and he would soon be sent to the SICU. I was aware that at times patients don't respond as well as expected, but I was comfortable in knowing that the intervention was immediate. Dr. Wojdylo's demeanor was very calm and he presented with no sense of concern, and we thanked him once more. Again, he said I could see Joe in about one hour.

After everyone was gone, Daneane and I sat in the lobby waiting to go upstairs to see Joe. More than an hour had passed and it was now about 3:45p.m. I went to the information desk to ask the attendant to check if we could see Joe. She called upstairs and spoke to someone in the recovery room, and we were told we couldn't see him yet. We sat and waited another 45 minutes, and it was now about 4:30 p.m. Again I went to the desk, and again she called upstairs and was told we could not go up yet. I told her that the surgeon said I would be able to see him in about an hour and it was now two hours. She stated this wasn't uncommon. She said, "The surgeons are always telling people they can go up sooner than they can, and everyone gets upset with me when they can't." I sat back down and waited once more, but now I could feel the anxiety building inside me.

It was now 5:10 p.m., and our son Joe had arrived at the hospital. Joe said, "Mom, his surgery was this morning, I can't believe you haven't seen him yet!" Joe was right. It was now 5:20, and it was going on three hours. I went back up to the desk, and this time I said to the attendant, "I want to see my husband right now, and if I can't I want a doctor down here in front of me this minute to tell me why not!" She then called upstairs and relayed my message to the party on the other end of the phone. We were then given permission to see him.

Outside the recovery room we were facing a large set of double doors. The surroundings were very quiet, and when the doors opened they made a very loud noise. Joe was in the first bed to the left inside the doors. When the doors opened, I could see his body from the chest down. With the noise of the doors his limbs suddenly jerked and stiffened toward the foot of the bed. It appeared that the loud noise had startled him, but then I was able to see his face. I was shocked! His eyes were wide open in a blank stare and his pupils appeared to be fixed and dilated, and his limbs remained very rigid. He appeared to have classic signs of brain damage. Immediately I looked at the cardiac monitors to see if his vital signs were stable. As I did, I could hear my son Joe scream, "Mom!" What's wrong with him?" Speechless, I looked at his nurse, who was by this time staring at me. Immediately she said "Oh he's ok, he's just so heavily sedated. In fact this is the first time he has even opened his eyes." As I looked back at Joe, his body relaxed, and his eyes closed as though he was sleeping again. I felt some relief, but his reaction to the noise was still causing some very deep concerns for me. I had never seen anyone coming out of anesthesia display such rigid movements. Patients are typically lethargic and difficult to arouse. I began to think that maybe he reacted like that because he was still intubated and not functioning on his own yet, but it had been over three hours, why wasn't he functioning on his own yet? Then remembered that Dr. Wojdylo said he was going to give him the extra pain medications. The nurse must have been right, the heavy sedation had to be the reason he was still asleep. I told our children he would be okay, and I sent them home. I told them I would stay until he was transferred to the SICU so I could talk to him once he woke up. They left, and I went back to the lobby to wait for his transfer.

I just couldn't shake the uneasy feelings of how Joe had reacted. I tried to convince myself that maybe I was over-reacting. Certainly Dr. Wojdylo would have told me if something were wrong. He was obligated to tell me, and he had already informed me that everything went well. Then why did I feel so much like something was wrong? I had to go back upstairs and see him again.

I went back to the desk, and the attendant called upstairs to tell them I was coming up again. I was told they were preparing him for his transfer to the SICU. I was then given directions to the SICU waiting room and told to go there and wait for him to arrive. I arrived in the waiting room at about 7:45 p.m. At approximately 8:00 p.m., I saw them wheeling Joe into the room. A nurse came and told me that as soon as they had him settled in she would come out and get me so I could visit with him. At approximately 8:20 p.m., while standing in the waiting room, I saw a man in scrubs coming down the hall towards me. He didn't look like a nurse, and I was the only one there, so I knew he was coming to speak to me. Suddenly I felt an overwhelming sense of dread. My heart started pounding hard in my chest, and my legs felt like they couldn't hold me up. As I sat down all I could think was "Please God, No!"

He introduced himself as Dr. Gray, the Chief Resident of the SICU. He sat in a chair across from me and said, "You know what happened don't you?" to which I replied "Nobody told me anything happened, why should I think that something did?" "Well, something did," he said, "At some point your husband lost all neurological function. He is starting to gain some of it back, but we don't know how much of it he will recover. We have scheduled a neurological consult for him to find out why this happened, but it will be midnight before the Neurologist will able to see Joe." I questioned him on the possibilities of what could have happened. He said they didn't know, but that they were in the process of trying to figure out what did. He said they were considering a possible stroke, bleeding in the brain, or the possibility of a blood clot, but they wouldn't know until after the neurological tests were completed. Dr. Gray also apologized for having to be the one to tell me. He said he was of the impression that someone had already spoken to me about it.

Why hadn't someone informed me of this before now? I had been there all day and evening, and the last doctor to whom Joe was delivered to for care, and the one who had nothing to do with the prior events of the day was the one left to tell me that something had happened. He was the doctor with the least amount of information.

I went in to see Joe, but he was still unresponsive. I just held his hand and talked to him. I begged him to wake up, and then demanded that he wake up. I was desperate for him to respond to me, and I felt like I was walking through a bad dream. Later that night I went home convinced that when I came back in the morning this would all be over, and everything would be fine. This really couldn't be happening.

When I arrived home I tried to tell our family what was happening. I didn't know how or what to tell them, as I myself didn't know. I could only say that Joe was not waking up, and nobody could tell us why. As I listened to the screams and the tears of our children, I myself couldn't cry. I felt that if I didn't cry, I wouldn't have to acknowledge that this was real.

I anxiously watched the clock until midnight and then called the hospital to see if the neurologist had examined Joe yet. I was told that Dr. Hollander had in fact examined him, and had ordered a CT scan of the brain. The CT scan would detect if there was any bleeding in his brain, or if a stroke had occurred. I was told to call back later for the results. I called back several times, and finally the answer was negative for both the stroke and the brain bleeding, but Joe remained unresponsive.

I called Dr. Gray several more times through the night, and most answers to my questions were vague. However, I was told that a heart attack was not a consideration for his condition, although Dr. Hollander did feel that something had happened that caused a major insult to Joe's brain. More tests would be needed in the morning. I was also informed that there was little documentation in Joe's chart to allow the medical staff to figure out what did happen. Then Dr. Gray stated, " What little documentation is there, is very unclear."

I felt as though I suddenly woke up. Anger took my attitude from that of a shattered wife to that of a trained medical professional. With all else ruled out, the only answer there could be was oxygen deprivation. Deprivation, long enough to cause severe brain damage. "Oh my God!" I screamed, "those bastards left him without oxygen long enough to destroy his brain, and now they're trying to cover up what they did!" They had even omitted information that was crucial for other doctors' who were following his care to have. This would delay them from finding out what had happened. I knew very well, that when something unforeseen happens to a patient in the course of a procedure, the family is immediately notified. Other doctors are then given a very detailed verbal report, and the documentation is always clear and precise, leaving nothing unexplained. In Joe's case, they were doing everything they could not to give an explanation. They had even tried to stop me from seeing him. They knew I was a nurse and would be able to identify that something was wrong with him, and they were not yet prepared with any answers they thought I would accept. It was now very obvious that an immediate response was not what Joe had received during his complication when his breathing tube was removed.

All the pieces were starting to fit, and I knew that something very wrong had taken place in that operating room. I wondered if Dr. Wojdylo knew when he came to see me, or if they had kept the truth from him as well. The questions were beginning to fire through my mind, and the pain and anger were unbearable. Now my tears were out of control. The only thing I knew for sure was that their lack of communication and unclear documentation made it very clear they were doing everything they could to keep whatever happened contained within the walls of that operating room. I needed to go back to the hospital immediately. Joe and Nick came with me.

CHAPTER III

When we walked into the SICU, Dr. Myers was standing on the right side of Joe's bed, and Dr. Wojdylo was on the left. They were both looking down on him, and both looked very perplexed. When I walked to the foot of Joe's bed, they turned to look at me. I said, "I want to know what happened to my husband, and I want to know right now!" As I spoke those words, I noticed a nurse standing behind Dr. Myers, and she was staring at me. Her facial expression was very serious, and as our eyes met, she squinted, and firmly nodded her head yes, as if telling me you'd better find out.

Dr. Wojdylo then asked me to go to a small office connected to the SICU. He said he would meet me there in a few minutes to explain. When he entered the room I could no longer contain myself. I screamed, "How could you talk to me so casually yesterday and lead me to believe nothing was wrong? How dare you do that to me! How long was he without oxygen? Dr. Wojdylo spoke in a very somber tone, "They told me he was reintubated immediately, I didn't know the extent of the damage until I saw Joe this morning." Nick firmly asked him again, "How long was he without oxygen?" He then stated that Dr. Proper, the anesthesiologist, and Dr. O'Malley, the surgical resident, had informed him that when Joe was extubated he appeared to develop what is called laryngospasms (the vocal cords lock together and cause the airway to obstruct), but that Dr. Proper had immediately re-established his airway. It wasn't until later when Joe wasn't able to wake up that Dr. Wojdylo questioned Dr. Proper again. This time he told Dr. Wojdylo that after Joe's airway had been re-established, they had proceeded to re-connect the monitors and found Joe's heart rate to be very slow. They were unable to feel a pulse, and CPR was initiated. Dr. Proper said that in his opinion Joe's heart must have gone into what is called electromechanical disassociation (EMD), a condition in which electrical signals are being sent, but the heart is not responding to the signal and is not pumping out the blood, thus causing cardiac arrest. Dr. Proper was claiming this as the possible cause of Joe's brain damage. Dr. Wojdylo could not get an answer from Dr. Proper regarding the length of time Joe was without oxygen. I said, "How can you find that explanation acceptable?" He replied "That's all the information I had to go by, I was down in the lobby with you when this happened."

As we left the office my pain and anger were now coupled with insult. This was an anesthesiologist who had obviously extubated my husband too soon, and then left him without oxygen long enough to cause severe brain damage and cause his heart to stop. He then failed to document any details of this event, and refused to verbalize any time frames of these events even to the surgeon. Now he was trying to claim that Joe's heart was the cause of his condition. First of all, Dr. Hollander had already ruled out Joe's heart as a possible cause of the damage to his brain. Secondly, why did Joe have to be reconnected to the monitors before they determined his heart was in trouble, why was he disconnected that soon after surgery in the first place? I kept telling myself to put my pain on hold and think with my head, and my head was telling me that something was very wrong here.

When we stepped into the hallway after leaving the office, Dr. Myers was standing there waiting for me. He expressed his sorrow, and said he was completely appalled with the entire situation. He then told me that he had briefly reviewed Joe's chart but had not been able to determine what had really happened. His plan was to further review the chart, and to talk to as many people as he could that were present in the OR to determine what had happened, and he would get back to me.

When Dr. Myers left, we were standing in the hall by ourselves. I could see that Joe and Nick were filled with the same pain and disbelief that I was. We then went in to see Joe. The sight of him was absolutely gut wrenching. He was on a respirator, and there were many lines connecting him to the monitors and the medications. His face and body were very swollen from the fluids he was receiving and the trauma he had undergone, and he was still unresponsive. The reality was overwhelming for all of us. This time I couldn't talk to Joe. This time I could only hold his hand and cry. We all remained silent and just cried.

CHAPTER IV

It was now late morning, and family and friends had started lining the hall outside of the SICU. As much as I appreciated the gestures of support, I just couldn't to talk to anybody. Our daughter Daneane, Joe's dad, his brother Nick and his sister Darlene had now arrived. I took them in to see Joe, and then made my way back to a corner of the waiting room where I had positioned myself earlier to avoid the crowd.

Dr. Myers returned. This time he informed me that he had completed an extensive review of Joe's chart, and could find nothing to explain Joe's condition. He said all information concerning the time of the event was either very poorly documented, or not documented at all. He had used the exact same words that Dr. Gray did when he had reviewed Joe's chart. Dr. Myers did locate one note written by Dr. O'Malley, and the note said, "Patient was extubated, quickly reintubated, heart rate decreased and no pulse palpable, CPR started with patient quickly responding to the cardiac medications given. Unlikely primary cardiac event." Dr. O'Malley was in that operating room, did he really think this was sufficient documentation for a man left in Joe's condition? This note was filled with what he was trying not to say.

All of the documentation followed in the same manner. Anything written by anyone present in the OR at the time of the event was very vague and lacked any details. The only thing that was clearly documented, was that each time a number on the record was written showing the time of Joe's extubation, the number 4 was written over it.

A short time later we learned that a meeting was called in the recovery room soon after Joe was transferred there. In attendance at this meeting was the medical staff from the OR at the time of the event, the medical staff in the recovery room, and some members from Hospital Administration. I suppose you wouldn't have to be a fly on the wall to know what was discussed at that meeting. Thus, the "Medical Code of Silence" began. Forget that your negligence has just destroyed a man's life. Forget the pain that his family is going through, and what they will have lost as a result of this. Forget that they at least deserve to know the truth and not be insulted with lies. Instead, they needed to do everything possible to cover their asses, and most importantly the hospital's ass. Ethics would not be practiced here.

Dr. Myers spent several hours reading Joe's chart and talking to everyone from whom he felt he might be able to get some information. There were never any answers. In fact, he told me that even after obtaining an explanation from Dr. Proper himself, what really happened was still very unclear.

It was now about 7:30 p.m. on Friday evening. I was sitting in the SICU waiting room with our family and some close friends. There were still some friends in the hallway outside the waiting room. The atmosphere was like that of a funeral parlor. My chest felt like there was a hole where my heart used to be, and I was going from heartache to anger, to fear, and confusion, over and over again. Now, some thirty hours after the event, Dr. Proper came walking into the waiting room. When he came in he introduced himself, then sat in a chair next to me and said, "I'm sorry I didn't get here sooner, but I've been busy." I could feel my stomach in my throat like I was going to vomit. Imagine being too busy to let a family know what had happened to their loved one while they were in your care. I thought, "The only thing he was busy doing was rehearsing what he was going to say to cover up what he had done." He said he wanted to give me an explanation of what had happened after Joe's surgery. After thirty hours and three doctors who could not get a straight answer from this man, he wanted to give me an explanation of what happened. Why in the name of God would I believe anything he had to say? At this point I really just wanted him out of my sight, and I couldn't look at him as he spoke to me. I just stared straight ahead while he proceeded to recite all the same words I had already heard from Dr. Wojdylo. When he was finished speaking, Joe's father who was hearing his story for the first time, spoke out and said "How long was Joe without oxygen?" It was at that point I did turn to look at him. That was the one answer he had been unwilling to document or give to any of the doctors who had asked him. He then stated, "Oh, three, four, five minutes tops," and immediately stood up and walked out of the room. He never once said that he was sorry for what had happened.

That evening after everyone left, I stayed in the waiting room. I desperately needed to sleep, but I just couldn't. I was exhausted, and each time I started to fall asleep, I would suddenly wake up. Each time I would go to Joe's bedside to check on him, but each time nothing had changed.

Saturday would give us a few more answers than the day before, but none of them were good, and Joe still remained unresponsive. Dr. Hollander, the neurologist, had ordered an EEG to be done that morning. The EEG would determine the amount of damage to Joe's brain. The results would either give us hope, or further tear our world apart. We would get an answer later in the day after Dr. Hollander was able to review the results of the test.

Before we were able to get the information from Dr. Hollander, yet another problem would occur. A pulmonary specialist informed me that Joe's lungs were now starting to show signs of failure. He said, "You're a nurse aren't you?" I replied," Yes, I am." He said, "Then I'm sure you know there are some moral issues that need to be addressed here." Hearing those words, I just about lost my mind. Clearly this man was suggesting that I place Joe on "Do Not Resuscitate" status. I hadn't even been given the details of his condition yet, how could he suggest I make a decision about his life! I just glared at him and said, "The only moral issue that I'm going to address here is how my husband went into that operating room for abdominal surgery, and came out brain damaged!" The doctor just walked away, but I remained quite shaken from what he had said.

It was now about 5:00 p.m., and Dr. Hollander had arrived to give us the test results. We gathered in the SICU waiting room. Our children and Joe's father were with me. Dr. Hollander stated that Joe had indeed suffered severe anoxic brain damage. The cause was a direct lack of oxygen to the brain for a prolonged period of time. He classified his condition as that of being in an "Alpha coma," and described the prognosis as "Lousy." He stated, " Nobody has ever come out of an alpha coma." He then explained that one of three things would happen, " Joe could get worse and then die, he could get a little better and then die, or he could remain the same and then die." Up until now I had clung to some hope that Joe would wake up and put an end to this nightmare. With Dr. Hollander's words, I felt that hope drain from inside me. Joe's dad asked him how long Joe would need to be without oxygen for this to happen. Of course Dr. Hollander stated there were too many variables for him to tell.

The scene in the room became very ugly. Everyone was crying, and then my son Joe started to become violent. He threw some chairs and kicked the garbage pail, and then started banging the walls with his fists. Nick grabbed him and held him until he stopped struggling, then they both just held each other and cried. Daneane and Joe's dad just sat in their chairs sobbing. I don't recall just how long we stayed in that room, but it felt like an eternity until the tears stopped flowing. For the first time in my life, I felt absolutely helpless. As a wife, I had to endure the pain of knowing I had lost my husband, knowing what he had suffered through, and knowing he was suffering still. As a mother, I had to endure the pain of watching my children suffering through the unbearable heartache of the loss of their father. There was nothing I could do to change either. Joe's dad was not a healthy man, and I also feared for his life, as I watched him struggle with the loss of his son.

Later that night after everyone left, I was sitting alone in the SICU waiting room when the wall phone rang. I couldn't imagine it was for me, but I was the only one there so I answered it. It was Joe's aunt Ester. Ester told me that she had just received a call from her daughter, Kathy Bellucco-Osborne. Kathy was attending a function in the Thousand Islands with her new husband and some of their friends. My first thought was, I really don't want to talk to anybody, and what does this have to do with me? I hadn't seen Kathy since my daughter's wedding in October of 1992. Then Ester proceeded to tell me that Kathy was telling some of her friends how upset she was that her cousin Joe had undergone surgery at Rochester General Hospital, and how he was now in a coma. As Kathy proceeded to tell the story as she thought it to be, she was suddenly interrupted by an acquaintance named Tammy Jo Higgins. Tammy suddenly announced, "That's not what happened," to which Kathy replied, "How do you know?" Tammy then stated, "Because I was there." Kathy then asked her to please tell her what really happened. Tammy stated she was currently employed as an anesthesia technician at Rochester General Hospital. Her job was to go into the operating rooms at the end of each surgery and replace and restock all of the used equipment and supplies on the anesthesia cart to prepare for the next surgery. That day Tammy and another anesthesia technician, under whom Tammy was training, named Debra Fader, were summoned to operating room # 4 where Joe was, to start the "Room turnover," as the cleaning of the room is called. Upon entering the room, Tammy went straight to the anesthesia cart to start taking inventory of the supplies she would need to replace. Debra went to the anesthesia machine and started stripping it of the old tubing. After several minutes, Tammy had completed her list and when turning to go to the stock room for the needed supplies, she noticed Joe lying on the hospital bed. She said that his face was blue. She thought this wasn't right, but not having any medical training, and the fact that nobody was near him or doing anything to him, she remained silent. She left the room and gathered her stock, returning several minutes later. When she entered the room this time, she said everyone was gathered around Joe and appeared to be working in a panic, and she could see that he was now dark blue. At that point, Debra Fader ran up to her and told her she would have to get out of there because she was just a student. She left the room, but remained upset the rest of the day from what she had seen. Debra later told Tammy that it was she who had noticed that Joe was dark blue, and when she did, she said, "Hey, is something wrong here, is this suppose to be this way?" It was only then that the medical staff in the room all ran to Joe's bedside.

Tammy stopped talking to Kathy at that point because Tammy's boyfriend Jason told her she had best "Shut-up." He reminded Tammy that she was supposed to keep all information about the patients confidential. Kathy immediately called her mother and said she wanted to repeat the conversation word for word quickly so she wouldn't forget any part of it. I thanked her for the information and we hung up. I so wished I had that information the night before when Dr. Proper sat before me with his big speech about how quickly he responded to Joe. I could have asked him if he started counting the minutes Joe was without oxygen before or after he turned dark blue. Maybe I could have just stood up and slapped him right across his pathetic lying face. Now I felt like I was choking with anger.

Sunday was a fairly quiet day. I did however receive a phone call from Dr. Myers, who was in the hospital and still searching for answers. He informed me that he had once again spoken with Dr. Proper, and this time Dr. Proper told him that Joe was without oxygen for about ten minutes. I informed him that on Friday Dr. Proper had told us it was "three, four, five minutes tops." Dr. Myers said he wanted me to know what Dr. Proper had said so I wouldn't hold on to any false hope for recovery. What difference did it make what Dr. Proper had said, he changed his times and story every time he spoke to somebody. By this time I knew I would never get the truth, and Tammy's story had confirmed why.

On August 20th we went forth with my son Joe's wedding. Of course we had reduced it to a small afternoon dinner with just family and a few very close friends. The day was filled with sadness and tears, and we could barely get through it. I told Joe that his father wasn't dead, and could remain as he was for very long time. The future was so uncertain, I felt it was best he go forward with his life. After the wedding I went back to the hospital. I couldn't compose myself as I told Joe the wedding was over. I had promised him so many times I would make sure he was there, and now I felt like I had betrayed him. I swore to him that if he ever woke up we would do it all over again and have a real wedding.

CHAPTER IV

Joe had encountered several complications during his stay in the SICU. He had to have the tube removed from this throat that connected him to the respirator, and they performed a tracheotomy on him. His surgical incision opened causing his intestines to protrude through his abdomen. He then had to be taken back into surgery to close the surgical incision a second time. He had also developed Pseudomonas in his lungs, which is a potentially deadly infection, often developed by patients who are on a respirator for a lengthy period of time. After two and a half weeks Joe was able to breathe on his own with just the help of oxygen. He was taken off the respirator and transferred to a room on the fourth floor. I had them put a lounge chair in his room that I could use as a bed for the remainder of his stay. I had no intention of leaving him there alone. In fact, I had already contacted Dr. Mary Dombovy at Saint Mary's Brain Injury Unit to see if I could have him transferred there. Dr. Dombovy told me he would have to be medically stable before a transfer would be considered. That didn't happen for another two months.

A couple of days after Joe's transfer to the forth floor, I was sitting in his room looking out at the nurse's station. Dr. Grunspan had finally returned from his vacation and was now standing there reading Joe's medical chart. I don't know why, but I felt a sense of comfort with him there. Dr. Myers had been absolutely wonderful, but

Dr. Grunspan had been our family doctor for more than seven years, and I was relieved that he was back. After reviewing the chart, he came into the room to examine Joe. He just stood there for several minutes looking at Joe and shaking his head. Then he looked at me and said, "What happened?" I immediately burst into tears. "They left him without oxygen until he was brain damaged, and now Dr. Proper is trying to blame it on his heart." In an effort to stop my tears, he walked to Joe's side, bent over and shouted in Joe's face, "Joe, the Giants suck!" With no response from Joe, he looked at me and said, "Yep, he's in trouble." He and Joe had a long history of bickering over their football teams. I stopped sobbing and smiled. I said, "Yes, he certainly is." He then told me he had reviewed the case with Dr. Myers and Dr. Wojdylo, and that there were several things he wanted done. He ordered another neurological consult with a Dr. Gilmore. Joe had not had any neurological follow up since the initial testing. He was also concerned about the statements regarding Joe's cardiac status, so he called Dr. Thompson, a cardiologist on the hospital staff, to do a complete evaluation of Joe's heart. This was partly to determine whether a cardiac event did take place, and partly to see if Joe's heart was something he needed to be concerned about for his future care. He also informed me that he was going to go to the Hospital Review Board and request that they set up a meeting with me, and give me the explanation that I deserved, about what happened.

These things would take place over the next few days, but the immediate concern was the fact that Joe had now developed very high fevers, around 106 degrees. These fevers were also causing his heart rate to increase up to 200 beats a minute. Dr. Grunspan was concerned that a rate that high could eventually cause his heart to give out. He had Joe transferred back to the SICU where he was put in a bed of ice to decrease his temperature. This was the intervention, the cause still needed to be determined. It was thought that the source of the elevated temperatures was core. Core, meaning that his brain would normally control his body temperature, but his brain was not functioning, therefore unable to do so. If that were the case, there would be nothing they could do. Temperatures that high would eventually kill him.

The following day Joe's temperature, although still elevated, was somewhat under control, and he was transferred back to his room on the fourth floor. The cardiologist was then able to start his evaluation. When Dr. Thompson arrived he reviewed Joe's chart, and then came into his room. He said, "Mrs. Nucci, can you tell me what happened? I can't figure it out from reading the chart. Of course you can't I replied, every doctor who has read Joe's chart has come in here to ask me what happened because they can't figure it out from the documentation in his chart, that's the way they want it. He then asked, "That's the way who wants it?" I said, "This hospital, and everybody who was in that operating room." There was no further conversation and he proceeded with his evaluation.

He reviewed Joe's cardiac history, previous and current EKGs, performed a physical exam, and followed with an echocardiogram. He then left to review the tests. He returned later that day. He said, "Mrs. Nucci, I've completed my examination and I want you to know that Joe's heart played no part in contributing to the condition of his brain. He did not, nor has he ever had a heart attack. I also want you to know that my documentation will clearly state as such." I thanked him from the bottom of my heart. Again I was beginning to feel overcome with anger. He had confirmed what I had known all along. Part of me was relieved to know I hadn't been wrong, part of me was angrier to know I hadn't been wrong. No matter what I felt, it still couldn't help Joe.

Dr. Gilmore, continued to follow Joe through the remainder of his hospital stay, ordering various tests and checking him everyday. Unfortunately there was very little change in his brain function. Although both Dr. Grunspan and Dr. Myers approached the Hospital Review Board several times to ask them to meet with me, they never did.

CHAPTER V

Joe remained at Rochester General Hospital for the next two months. During his stay he battled one infection after another. He had also developed an abscess in his abdomen near his surgical incision that had to be drained. More infection, more antibiotics, more elevated temperatures, and some irregular breathing patterns suggestive that death may be imminent. Joe endured a long hard battle, but through it all his heart remained very strong.

At the end of two months, there was nothing more that could be done for Joe. He was as medically stable as he was ever going to be, and it was time for him to be discharged from the hospital. This couldn't come a minute too soon as far as I was concerned. I had taken family leave from my job, and stayed with Joe around the clock. Our children, and Joe's dad, brother, and sister came to see him daily. Everybody's life was turned upside down, but the hardest part of being in that hospital was controlling the animosity that each of us felt. Even after two months, conversations still went silent if we approached any staff as they were talking. The nurses still sheepishly stared at us, and were very careful about their choice of words when having to speak with us, which they kept as limited as possible. The situation was stressful for everyone, and I'm sure they were as happy to see us leave as we were to go. Nobody wanted to say anything wrong knowing they could lose their job if they did. After all, Tammy Higgins had been terminated one week after her conversation with Kathy Bellucco-Osborne.

I was very anxious to get Joe transferred to the Brain Injury Unit at St. Mary's Hospital, but this would not be an easy task. Again I called Dr. Dombovy to request the transfer. She said someone from her practice would come to evaluate Joe for placement there, but that they rarely, if ever, accepted patients with brain damage caused by anoxia. There was really nothing that could be done for these patients. I wished she had told me this the first time I called her. For the past two months my heart was set on having him transferred there. I wanted to give Joe every possible chance available for recovery.

Joe was evaluated by one of Dr. Dombovy's associates, Dr. Orsini. Dr. Grunspan notified me that according to the note Dr. Orsini had documented in Joe's medical chart, Joe was not accepted for placement. I was heart broken. I was so hopeful that with professional therapy Joe might be able to recover some awareness or function. Now I would never get the opportunity to find out.

Dr. Grunspan came to talk to me about what our next step should be. He suggested that I place Joe in a nursing home. We had to leave Rochester General, and St. Mary's wouldn't take him, but the thought of letting him rot to death in a nursing home was not one I was even willing to entertain. If Joe had any chance for some recovery, as little as it may be it certainly wouldn't be in a place where he could be treated like a dead piece of meat. I told Dr. Grunspan, "He's my husband, and he's been through enough, he isn't going anywhere but home." I knew that providing Joe with the constant care that he needed would involve big sacrifices for me, but they were sacrifices I was willing to make. Dr. Grunspan asked me to think my decision through very carefully. I already did, the day I stood in front of God and took my wedding vows. They had included, "In sickness and in health." Dr. Grunspan would begin making the arrangements to have him transferred home

As I sat at Joe's bedside, I was filled with fear about the uncertainty of my life. After all this time, this still felt like a very bad dream. I continued to feel that some day Joe was going to wake up and this would all be over. Someday we would continue with our lives as we had planned.

It was now about 5:30 p.m., and the phone in Joe's room rang. The voice on the other end said, "Hello Linda, this is Mary Dombovy calling." I wasn't surprised to hear her voice, because I had called her earlier in the day and left a message with her secretary to have her to call me back. I wanted her to accept Joe at St. Mary's, and I was prepared to beg her if I had to, but I never did. She proceeded to tell me that she had changed her mind and had decided to accept Joe. I was to meet with her the next day to tour the unit at St. Mary's, and to review what was expected of me. She would have Joe transferred there the following day, but she made it very clear that he could only stay there for a couple of weeks while they trained me to care for a brain injured person. While he was there, he would receive the benefits of further tests and therapy. I asked her what had changed her mind. She said the fact that I insisted on taking him home. I didn't really care why, I had accomplished my goal, and Joe's foot was now in the door.

CHAPTER VI

When Joe arrived at St. Mary's, Dr. Dombovy came into his room to examine him. She kept looking back and forth examining his eyes and then his limbs, and making notes. She appeared to be confused, and she then called several other doctors into the room to examine him as well. I asked her what was wrong. She said she wasn't sure, more tests would be needed in the morning, but she felt there was something more neurological going on with him. She said he showed signs of a possible spinal injury. I said "Instead of anoxia?" She stated, "No, besides the anoxia." "Do you think they may have dropped him too?" I said, "How else could he sustain a spinal injury?" She just stated that his symptoms were very confusing, and Joe would need several more tests before she could reach any conclusions.

One day during Joe's stay, Dr. Dombovy came into his room and told me that she was now playing phone tag with a Dr. Proper at Rochester General. She asked me if I knew who he was. I told her who he was, and then stated "Don't bother calling him back, he probably just wants to know if you figured out what he did." I found it odd that she didn't recognize his name, but I didn't question her about it, I thought maybe she had simply forgotten it. I would find out several years later in court why she didn't know who he was.

While at St. Mary's, Joe underwent numerous tests and very aggressive physical, speech, and occupational therapy. Some of the test results appeared encouraging, and some were not so encouraging. Sometimes during therapy it would appear he was right on the edge of breaking through, and sometimes the effort would appear completely worthless. Everyday was emotionally draining. His prognosis was changed several times, but at the end of six weeks I took him home in pretty much the same condition as when we had arrived. Dr. Dombovy was never able to rule out or confirm a spinal injury.

CHAPTER VII

November 23rd 1994, we took Joe home. The coming years would be a living hell for our entire family. The magnitude of destruction this tragedy had caused was unimaginable. Joe's care was never ending, as was the agony of seeing him in this condition every day. The laughter in our house was now replaced with heavy hearts, and daily tears and sadness. Every day our children would spend time with their father touching him and talking to him, hoping that something they would say or do would evoke a response from him. Every day the frustration of no response would evoke a deeper sadness in them. I could literally see their hearts ache. It was like watching life draining from them, a little more each day. It was a feeling I knew all too well, but it was not one I could accept for them.

Watching our grandchildren, Johnathan and Kayci was also incredibly painful. Joe was their fun, and loving Papa, and they were the sunshine of his life. They had a very special relationship with him. He would spend many hours playing with them, and no matter how naughty they would be, they were his "Golden children" and could do nothing wrong. He was also their protector, and whenever their parents punished them for doing something wrong, they would retaliate by saying "I'll tell Papa." Joe of coarse had gotten a big kick out of this. When I would tell Joe to stop interfering with their need for discipline, he would say, "When I was young it seemed I was working all the time and I missed so much of watching our own children grow. I feel like God has given me a second chance."

Kayci had now become very protective of Joe. Although she was only two years old, every time someone would visit Joe she would run to the chair in the corner of his room and just sit there and watch them. If they spoke to him she would immediately say "Papas tired, he can't talk now." I don't know what was in her little mind, but it was painful watching her make excuses for Joe's silence. We didn't know if she really believed what she was saying. If she didn't then what kind of emotional upset was this child going through? If she did, what would happen in time when she realized the truth? The potential long-term effects on her were frightening.

Johnathan, who was eight at the time, had a little more understanding of the situation. He would just sit and stare at Joe. Sometimes he would cry and sometimes he wouldn't. Often I would find him standing next to Joe's bed just touching him. I would encourage him to talk to his grandfather, but he refused. One day I said, "Johnathan, lets pray for Papa together, maybe God will help him, they say he listens to children." His response was painful, and his anger was obvious. He said, "Don't lie to me Grandma, you know he isn't going to get better." I didn't know if encouraging him to hold on and believe was the right thing to do, so I told him "No matter what happens, just remember Papa loves you very much, and always will." Johnathan is now sixteen years old, and still on occasion we find him just standing silently, staring at Joe and crying. He has never talked to his Grandfather.

Joe loved those children so much, and their lives had now been stripped of the benefits of their Grandfather's love, and he theirs. I wished for nothing but pain and loss in the lives of everyone in that operating room. I wanted them to experience and feel what their negligence had taken from us. I couldn't stand the thought that they could go on with their lives without feeling what they had done to ours. I wanted them wake up everyday with the same never-ending pain in their hearts that we had to live with. I don't now, nor will I ever, forgive any of them.

I had to return to work as I was soon headed for financial demise. I had exhausted all of our life savings during Joe's hospital stay. The medical insurance would only provide a very limited amount of nursing hours, and family had to provide most of his care. I was able to return to work part time, by working two sixteen-hour days a week. This was physically difficult for me, and my financial future was not looking very bright, but those were the least of my concerns at that time. Just making it through each day was the biggest. My children took care of their father while I was working, and I spent the other five days of the week caring for him myself. Their support was incredible, and I know I couldn't have survived without it, but seeing them taking on such a tremendous burden made me sick with guilt. They were so young, yet they were making sacrifices with their lives that most adults wouldn't be willing to make. I would often tell them how badly this made me feel, to which they would respond, 'He's our dad, we love him too." I was so proud of them. The beauty of it was that they loved him that much. The sadness of it was that they loved him that much.

I tried to stay focused on Joe, and on providing him with the best chance of recovery that I could possibly give him. I had physical, speech, and occupational therapists, working with him. I had even hired a music therapist. The insurance ran out on the therapy coverage, but I had watched each one of the therapists as they had worked with him, so I could continue giving him the therapy myself after they were gone. I spent month after month working with Joe each day as long as I could physically endure. I would still wake up every morning and go to his bedside thinking maybe today will be the day he speaks to me. Maybe today he'll answer me when I talk to him. Maybe today he'll say my name or even just hello. Those were my thoughts each morning, and by the end of each day my disappointment would reduce me to tears.

Dr. Dombovy told me that I needed to change my expectations. She said I had to think in terms of months and years, not days. She was right, and after approximately two years had passed, Joe started to cry whenever I would talk or sing to him. His response was very slow at first. He would only cry once every few weeks. He then cried weekly, and eventually daily. He would also respond to our children's voices with tears. At first I was very happy and excited. I kept waiting for his next response, wondering what it would be and when it was going to happen. This gave me the strength that I needed to keep going, and I prayed all the time. I kept thinking that God wouldn't take him this far and not keep going. There had to be a reason he was keeping Joe alive.

Eventually Joe was able to blink twice on command. Because he could never do this on a consistent basis, the doctors felt it wasn't purposeful or voluntary. I believed it was voluntary, but that his responses were just delayed. Even when Joe wasn't able to quickly respond, his expression was that of someone deep in thought, as though he were trying to process what he had been told. Many of Joe's facial expressions were the same as they were before this had happened. I was the one that was with him everyday, and I used those facial expressions to determine many of his needs. I wasn't trying to be unrealistic, but I was convinced that he was able to process some thoughts. Joe simply lacked the ability to communicate those thoughts. His doctors would spend ten minutes looking at him once a year, and then opine that he had no sense of awareness. I understood their opinion based on what they were seeing, but I wanted them to acknowledge what I saw in him as well.

One day I made a video of Joe during one of his crying episodes and then sent the tape to Dr. Dombovy. A couple of days later, Dr. Dombovy called to tell me she had scheduled Joe for a Stimulus EEG with Dr. Berg at Strong Memorial Hospital. She felt it was necessary that she have another neurologist do the testing. She acknowledged that she may be too close to the situation, and because of this her opinions may be biased.

A Stimulus EEG involved monitoring Joe's brain while providing various forms of stimulus when recording his reactions. At the completion of the test, Dr. Berg concluded that although Joe did show some noted improvement in the higher learning center of his brain, it was not enough to change his prognosis or for him ever to become functional. Once again our hopes were shattered.

Each disappointment was getting harder to overcome than the one before. Each one made me feel like I was losing another piece of my heart. This time I found myself questioning my faith in God.

What did he want from me, and how much more of myself could I give before he would give Joe back to us. Each day in my prayers I would beg him for the miracle that I knew only he could give us. I believed that he had kept Joe alive because he had a plan unbeknown yet to me. I also believed that if I kept my faith and did my part he would reward Joe and give him back his mind. I was afraid not to believe, but now I could feel my faith slipping away. My prayers became demanding, and now when I prayed I would say "God, either take him or give him back to us, but don't leave him like this any longer." As time passed, I began to believe that either God didn't care, or he just didn't exist.

I stopped looking for reasons to hold on, and I was now looking for reasons to let go. This wouldn't happen, as I couldn't ignore the signs that Joe clearly maintained some sense of awareness. Could he be locked in a never-ending hell? Could this be why his only reaction was to cry? The frustration of not knowing and the thought of what he might be suffering through made me feel ill. All of the excitement we had experienced when seeing his reactions was now filled with regret. Now I hoped that if he couldn't come back, he didn't posses any sense of awareness at all, for his own sake.

Life was filled with a constant and deep emptiness. Our grieving was very different than that of a death. It felt like we were attending his funeral every day, yet we couldn't bury him and move forward to the next step of the grieving process. There was no closure in sight, and after four years, there was still no relief from the hate and the anger that filled me. I would often have thoughts of holding a plastic bag over Dr. Proper's head so I could watch him gasp for air while he turned dark blue. I wanted him to experience what five minutes without oxygen felt like. Never in my life have I ever had thoughts of harming anyone, and now I thought about it everyday. These feelings had to end, or I knew I would self-destruct.

CHAPTER VIII

I had initiated a lawsuit against Dr. Proper and Rochester General Hospital at the time of Joe's discharge from the hospital. I couldn't let them destroy our lives and just walk away from what they had done. I wanted Dr. Proper held accountable, and I refused to accept all the lies and the conspiracy that the hospital had obviously engaged in. The trial was now coming near, and I had been meeting with my attorney, Angelo Faraci, once a week for the past two months. During these meetings we would review all of the events prior to, during, and after the surgery. Mr. Faraci also needed to get to know me personally, as well as my family and my relationship with Joe. Everything would be put on trial. Angelo would say, "Just tell the truth, you can never go wrong with the truth." The truth was that I could remember every single detail as though it happened the day before. The problem was that verbalizing the details to him made me feel like it was happening all over again. This was very painful, and each session with him made me very emotional. I began to worry if I would be able to hold up in court. Hell, I couldn't even hold myself together in his office.

Our last meeting was on Monday, March 23rd, 1998. Jury selection was to begin on Thursday, and the trial would start the following Monday, March 30th. During the jury selection, It appeared that the defense was trying to dismiss anyone with any medical knowledge or background. It was obvious that they didn't want anyone on the jury that could understand what happened. I was relieved when we were able to keep a Nurse Practitioner.

I had waited four agonizing years for this trial, and now it was here. I knew I would never begin to heal until I could see them held responsible for what they had done to Joe, and for how much we were suffering. I believed in truth and justice, and once again I turned to my faith. I believed that if God did exist, he wouldn't let them get away with this. I felt confident that the truth would prevail, but I really wanted this to be over. Just the thought of having to be in the same room and look at those people from Rochester General made me sick. I didn't want to breathe from the same air as Dr. Proper. I realized that this was going to be a very grueling experience, and it was.

Monday morning, March 30th 1998, I walked into the courtroom with Mr. Faraci and a young attorney from his firm, John Falk. Michelle Callan, another attorney from the firm who had participated in the research of the case, and who had served as a great support for me personally, was also present. I suddenly felt overwhelmed and I could feel my heart racing in my chest. When all was settled in the courtroom, the court officer said "All rise" and we stood as Judge Syracuse entered the courtroom and took his chair at the bench. As I was looking at the Judge, my eyes caught the words written across the bench in front of him. They read, "In God We Trust." As I gazed at the words, I began to feel a strange sense of comfort. I thought; "This is where all of their lies' will end and the truth will be exposed." I was confident that no one could lie while under oath in a court of law."

After the Judge gave the jury instructions, opening statements began. Mr. Faraci was first, and he gave the jury a brief review of the evidence, how and why things happened as they did, the impact of Joe's condition on our lives, and how the defense attorneys would claim that Dr. Proper had done nothing wrong.

Mr. Brown, attorney for Dr. Proper, recited all of Dr. Proper's credentials. He stated that although this was a very sad case the jurors should not let their emotions get involved when deciding their verdict, and if Dr. Proper did do something wrong he should be found responsible, but of course, he had done nothing wrong.

Mr. Fox, attorney for Rochester General Hospital, wanted to stress what a wonderful and successful hospital they were, what a brilliant and well trained staff they had, and what a fat, worthless, drunken bum my husband was. And by the way, although they supported Dr. Proper's plea of not responsible, he definitely was not employed by the hospital, and therefore, they weren't responsible for his conduct. This guy came out of the gate rolling in the mud, and I didn't think there was room to go any lower. Angelo had warned me that I would hear many comments during the trial that would anger and hurt me, but that I would have to endure them.

I was the first to testify. It seemed like I was on the stand forever. Angelo asked me questions starting from the beginning of my marriage up to and through all the events at the hospital, and to the present. I felt like I was under a microscope, but I opened my life before everyone, with complete honesty. We then discussed each conversation that I had with each doctor while at the hospital, much to the objections of the defense attorneys on the grounds of hearsay, but the doctors were present to testify, so the Judge overruled each objection. We also presented a video of Joe so the jury could see him in his present condition, and I talked them through his daily care as we had filmed it on the video. At the completion of the video I was surprised and touched to see Judge Syracuse wiping his eyes. Then Angelo asked me how taking care of Joe made me feel. It was the one question I couldn't answer without falling apart. I struggled to put words together that would make some sense, but I just ended up bursting into tears. How could I possibly explain everything I had felt over the past four years? How could any words describe the heartache, the grief, the emptiness, anger, hate, frustration, and repeated disappointments I had to endure? Unless someone has been in my world, they could never understand the sadness that I lived in. We then took a short recess so I could regain my composure, and then I returned to the witness stand.

Mr. Brown questioned me next. He was brief, and only asked me if I had seen Dr. Proper become emotional and start to cry the day he came into the SICU waiting room to tell me what had happened. Of course he failed to mention that it took Dr. Proper over thirty hours before he offered me that explanation. How insensitive of me not to notice Dr. Proper's emotional state while he was trying to lie about how he had destroyed my husband's life, and how he was too busy to come and tell me about it. If I knew he was crying, that would have made it all okay.

Mr. Fox was not as brief, and his questions were as follows:

Q) Now in terms of your husband's medical history before August of 1994, I think you testified that he had an alcohol problem for some period of time for a few years during the time he had his restaurant?

A) No. What I said is that he had a problem from alcohol. He did not have an alcohol problem. There was never an addiction. He did however have some medical complications as a result of drinking excessively.

Q) He was using it daily, is that correct?

A) Yes, he was drinking daily except for Sundays.

Q) Multiple amounts each day?

A) I would have to think so; he was there for long hours.

Q) And he had high blood pressure?

A) As a result of the alcohol, yes.

Q) And he was a two pack a day smoker?

A) Correct.

Q) And he was about five foot seven, is that his height?

A) Yes.

Q) And he weighed about two hundred forty pounds or so?

A) He was two hundred and ten.

Q) Before the procedure?

I wanted to say was, he weighed as much before the procedure when Dr. Proper had assessed him as he did during the procedure. He didn't suddenly blow up on the OR table. His size as well as his smoking should have been a consideration before he was extubated. Dr. Proper could have had the janitor assess him if he wasn't going to use the information. But I maintained my composure and said: " The year before he had lost just under fifty pounds. He had been on a diet."

This was Mr. Fox's entire line of questions. One sling of mud after another, focused on trying to make Joe look bad. I was hoping the jury could see through what he was trying to do, and would also wonder, as I did, what Joe's history ten years prior to this incident had to do with anything. Furthermore, was he trying to suggest that if Joe wasn't a perfect person it was okay that this happened to him? Maybe if you're overweight you should expect to come out of surgery brain damaged, after all, it's your own fault isn't it? I suppose if you lack a credible defense, you can always attack the victim. It quickly became very obvious why he represented Rochester General Hospital; they both shared the same lack of integrity.

In 1984 Joe had opened a restaurant. It was something he had always dreamed of doing. Joe owned the restaurant from 1984 to 1987, working up to sixteen hours a day, six days a week. Many friends would frequent the restaurant to see Joe and share a drink with him. Because of the nature of the business, Joe was drinking alcohol on a daily basis. After three years the drinking and the lack of rest from the long hours he was working, had started to take a toll on Joe's health. He wasn't feeling well, and had developed high blood pressure as a result of the stress and alcohol consumption. Joe tried to take in a partner to give him some relief and some time away from the business, but when he was not successful in doing so, we both agreed for his health's sake he should close the restaurant, and he did. Joe had never developed an addiction to the alcohol. In fact Joe had said that after the past three years, the thought of putting another drink in his mouth made him sick. Now Mr. Fox was trying to portrait Joe as a degenerate fat alcoholic. This guy made my skin crawl.

At the end of my testimony, Mr. Faraci presented a timeline of events that had been extracted from Joe's medical records as well as from the sworn depositions of the witnesses' before the trial, especially from Dr. Proper's deposition. This timeline was presented on a large drawing board and was put together by a Legal Nurse Consultant, Claudia Egan, a former employee of Mr. Faraci's, who had assisted him in our case. The timeline would provide the jury with a clear picture of the timing and sequence of the events as they had taken place in the OR, and would clarify any discrepancies in the testimony of the witnesses. The operating room records themselves had also been enlarged for the jury to see, and clearly showed that the documents contained false information, as well as how many of the times on the documents had been very boldly written over. The significance of both, were a key factor in proving their neglect. Mr. Fox and Mr. Brown fought vigorously to keep this timeline from the jury. They literally wasted a whole afternoon to argue against letting Mr. Faraci present it, along with Claudia's testimony. The arguments actually carried into the next morning when it was decided the timeline would be put on hold for the time being. We were however, able to present the enlarged operating room documents.

On March 31st, the first witness was Dr. Joshua Hollander, the neurologist who had examined Joe in the SICU. Dr. Hollander was sworn in and Angelo reviewed his credentials. Dr. Hollander stated that he was Chief of Neurology at Rochester General and had maintained that position since 1969. He also taught neurology to medical residents and students.

Angelo proceeded with his questioning.

Q) Do you recall how it is that you came to see this patient?

A) I was asked to see the patient, and I didn't note who asked me. I assume it was either the surgical intensive care unit staff, which would be most likely, or perhaps Dr. Wojdylo.

Q) Doctor, when you arrived, do you have some memory of his appearance?

A) Yes. I remember someone with a very distended abdomen, and as I recall it was a large man.

Q) Was he neurologically unresponsive and on a respirator when you arrived?

A) Yes.

Q) Tell us briefly, what did you do on your examination and what findings did you make?

A) He had normal movement reflexes when you turned his head, and his face was symmetric. As I was examining him the tone changed from someone who was flaccid to someone who had increased tone and extension. Namely, his arms were straight out, not bent at the elbow.

Q) Was this change significant at all?

A) I think the two findings would imply different levels of the nervous system being involved, and that was a source of confusion for me as to what was going on.

My thoughts immediately flashed back to Dr. Dombovy's examination of Joe, and her statement "Something else neurological is going on." I was now convinced they had also dropped him, and caused him to sustain a spinal injury, but without sufficient evidence to support that, I needed to let those thoughts go.

Angelo:

Q) Go on please, complete your examination and findings on that examination.

A) Well, that basically he had no muscle strength, reflexes, no knee jerk or ankle jerk or biceps, and I thought that he had had some major intracranial disaster. I wasn't sure of the exact nature of that, and I suggested a CT scan to look at his brain.

Q) When you say your impression was he may have sustained an intracranial disaster, in lay terms, what were you thinking, what does that mean?

A) I thought that his posturing was indicative of the fact that the upper portions of his brain were not functioning, and that he was operating primarily from the brain stem responses, and that was bad. I wasn't sure exactly where in the brain stem we were, but this would mean some major insult to the brain had occurred.

Q) You didn't know in what portions of the brain that damage might be at that time, and you decided to do further tests in order to define what the problem was in the brain?

A) Yes.

Q) Now, what were the tests you ordered, why did you order them, and what did they show?

Dr. Hollander then explained that he had ordered a CT scan of the brain. The possibilities for Joe's condition that he was considering were, a bleeding into portions of his brain, an obstructed flow of spinal fluid, or a blockage in the basliar artery of his brain, which would indicate a stroke. His last consideration was that his brain had been deprived of oxygen for a sufficiently long period of time, and that was called anoxic encephalopathy.

Angelo:

Q) At some point did you form the diagnosis here in this case of severe anoxic encephalopathy?

A) Yes.

Q) Did you do that by the next day when you got the CT scan back and the results of that test?

A) Yes, and that was reinforced by subsequent evolution and additional testing.

Q) If you're reading the chart for information, what it tells you is that at 1:30, the monitors are not being charted and there is no oxygen being given thereafter; is that a fair statement?

A) There is no monitoring on the record; I don't have in this sheet any information about what the patient's oxygenation is.

Q) According to this chart, oxygen is not being delivered to this patient by the anesthesiologist. Is that fair? According to what you see on the chart, there isn't any more air or oxygen being given after 1:30, is that true?

A) There is no record on this sheet of what happened after that.

Q) For example, at one o'clock he's being given 37% oxygen, and at one thirty he's being given 38% oxygen, and then it stops, doesn't it?

A) The record stops.

Q) Now look down, if you would, to the note right down towards the bottom, you see where it says 1345?

A) Yeah.

Q) By the way, has that 45 been written over another number?

A) It's very hard to read. I'm not entirely clear. There are lines and the two numbers, but the minute numbers are not particularly legible to me.

Q) I haven't asked you what number is written under, but can you see that the number 45 has been written over something else?

A) I can't tell what I'm looking at, it's too badly written. I guess it depends on whether it's a 5 or a 3.

Q) Now, please turn to Dr. O'Malley's note of the same day. I take it in your review, when you were at the bedside and you were interested to know what had gone on, that would have been one of the records you reviewed, is that right?

A) Right.

Q) By the way, is the 4 written over another number?

A) Yes, the 4 is obviously written over something, which I'm not sure about.

Q) Does the note say: As the patient was moved to ICU bed, then extubated, he desaturated oxygen, meaning that he started losing oxygen in his blood?

A) Right.

Q) He says: EKG leads reconnected, and patient found to have rhythm of sinus bradycardia. What is that?

A) Slow heartbeat emanating from the normal conducting system.

Q) Now, the next thing that was determined was that the pulses were not palpable, is that correct?

A) Yes, the blood was not flowing to a level capable of causing pulses.

Q) So isn't it clear to you that the breathing problem came first, but they never were aware of a heart problem?

A) I guess that is right.

Q) Turn to the perioperative flowsheet, and turn to the second page. 1345, that's a note written by Nurse Linda Moore, is it not?

A) Yes.

Q) She has a short description that follows timing at 1345, is that correct?

A) Yes.

Q) Again, has the 4 been written over another number?

A) Yes.

Q) Can you tell what the number is underneath?

A) It's either a 5 or a 3.

Q) So this was changed from 1335 or 55 to 1345, is that what the record seems to show?

A) That's right.

Q) Would it be important for you to know how long he's been without oxygen in order to judge its effects, not only on the brain, but also on the heart?

A) I would need to know the severity and the duration, yes.

Q) Did you look in that record for any evidence regarding the duration that this patient was without oxygen during the period of time that the obstruction was determined and the period of time reintubation and ventilation was re-established?

A) I couldn't tell.

Q) But you did look for that information, didn't you doctor?

A) Yes.

Although Dr. Hollander was testifying honestly, it was obvious that he was not exactly comfortable giving the information that Angelo was getting from his answers. Although employed by the hospital, he was still not willing to compromise his integrity and reputation by giving false testimony. However, he seemed somewhat disturbed to learn there were so many times changed, that the record was beginning to look like a bad joke. Then Dr. Hollander located a note in the chart written by Dr. Proper. Excuse me, he told Angelo, you asked me about the severity which I didn't know, but there is an answer to that. Dr. Proper's note stated that the oxygen saturation was not less than 75 to 80%. Angelo jumped on this statement like it was a gift.

Angelo:

Q) Now how would you measure oxygen saturation?

A) This would be done by an external or internal device.

Q) You said it tells you how long he'd been without oxygen?

A) It doesn't tell me how long, but it tells me that the severity was not profound, because he never dropped below 70 or 80%.

Q) Do you accept that? With this man's condition, do you accept that the oxygen saturation never dropped below 75 to 80%?

A) That's all I have.

Q) Well, how is the oxygen saturation taken?

A) I don't know what device they might have used in this case.

Q) If they put that sensor on the ear or finger, that sensor is detecting blood flow isn't it? And the value of the oxygen saturation depends whether or not blood is circulating at the time you take it, right?

A) Yes.

Q) When they reconnected the EKG leads on this man right after they reintubated him, they found there was no blood flow, and no pulses, is that right?

A) Yes.

Q) And if this man had little or no blood flow, he couldn't get an oxygen saturation value, could he?

A) That's correct.

Cross-examination by Mr. Brown began.

Q) Doctor, when you came in on 8/11/94, you saw this patient in the PACU?

A) No, in the Surgical Intensive Care Unit.

Q) And that's where you did your examination?

A) Yes.

Q) And any information contained in that record concerning events that occurred prior to your arrival was obtained by a review of certain records, is that correct?

A) That's correct.

Q) So, that information that follows is the information you got from Dr. O'Malley's note of that time?

A) Right.

Q) If the time was anything else you would have written something else in there, and any information you put in your record that preceded your involvement in this case would be information you gleaned from reviewing other records that were present at the time?

A) Yes. Mr. Brown: That's all I have, thank you. Mr. Fox: Your Honor, I have no questions for Dr. Hollander.

I was really confused as to the significance of Mr. Brown's questions, but that thought was brief. I was really more impressed with the fact that with one witness, Angelo was able to establish that without question Joe's condition was caused by lack of oxygen to the brain for a lengthy period of time, and that his heart was not a contributing factor to this condition. He had also established that the times on his record were clearly altered to close the gap of the time from extubation to reintubation, and that information contained in Dr. Proper's note regarding Joe's oxygen status was absolutely false.

The next witness was Dr. Wojdylo, the surgeon. Once again Mr. Faraci started by reviewing Dr. Wojdylo's credentials, and his status with the hospital. They also reviewed Joe's admission, the coarse of care that was initially taken, and then moved on to Joe's need for surgery.

Mr. Faraci:

Q) There came a time, that Mr. Nucci's condition of diverticulitis began to worsen and he showed signs of obstruction?

A) Yes. Dr. Meyers asked me to consult on Mr. Nucci to see him for his diverticulitis, and see if there would possibly in the future be any need for surgery. When I first examained him there was not, and the treatment with the antibiotics and bowel rest, nothing to eat, was appropriate. Over the next several days after I saw him, he gradually became increasingly distended, that was, his belly began to swell up, he had more pain, and he had some x-ray signs of increasing distension and early obstruction.

Q) Now, did there come a time before August 11th that you examined him and recommended surgery?

A) Yes.

Q) Surgery occurred on August 11th, and in surgery we have had some evidence that Dr. Proper was the anesthesiologist, and you were the surgeon?

A) Yes.

Q) Linda Moore was the circulating nurse?

A) Yes, I believe so.

Q) Now in addition to those individuals, was there also a Dr. O'Malley on the team?

A) Yes. He was one of the surgical residents.

Q) What does that mean?

A) He's a physician who's still in training to become a surgeon. He was to assist me with the surgery.

Q) Surgery took what, some four hours, and it was unexpectedly long?

A) It was a little longer than normal because of removing the right part of the colon, so it's probably an hour more than originally expected.

Q) During surgery, what was the role of Dr. Proper?

A) He's responsible for keeping the patient asleep and relaxed, and maintaining the patient's airway.

Q) How would he do that?

A) Through an endotracheal tube.

Angelo had Dr. Wojdylo explain that an Endotracheal tube is the breathing tube that is placed into a patient's airway before surgery starts, and that it was used during surgery to administer the drugs to anesthetize the patient as well as to administer air and oxygen throughout the procedure. He also explained that patients were unable to breathe on their own during surgery, because the anesthetics they receive paralyzed their respiratory function.

Angelo:

Q) With respect to the anesthesia record, does it show that during the surgery Forane was given as part of the drugs?

A) Yes.

Q) What is Forane, and does it affect brain function?

A) Forane is a general anesthetic that keeps the patient asleep. That's what sedates the brain.

Q) As far as Forane is concerned it was administered at what time?

A) One o'clock.

Q) And what does Norcuron do?

A) Norcuron is a paralyzing agent. It paralyzes the muscles.

Q) And Norcuron was administered initially six milliliters at ten o'clock, and then another four milliliters between 11:30 and 11:45, and then another two milliliters between 11:45 and 12:00. A) Yes.

Q) Then FOUR milliliters 15 minutes before the end of the procedure?

A) Yes.

I couldn't believe what I was hearing! Obviously the doses of this paralyzing agent were being titrated down from the beginning of surgery, so why on earth would he be given a larger dose 15 minutes before the end of surgery? If two milliliters held him from 12:00 to 1:15, how could he possibly receive four milliliters fifteen minutes before the completion of the surgery and be expected to function without assistance? This was beginning to sound criminal. Sedating his brain, paralyzing his muscles, and then within a brief period of 15 minutes removing his breathing tube went far beyond neglect.

Mr. Faraci continued:

Q) Did Mr. Nucci come through surgery successfully, was everything okay.

A) Up to that point in time, yes.

Q) Did you and Dr. Proper discuss the length of the surgery and it effects or possible effects on the patient?

A) Yes. We discussed the surgery had been a while, several hours, and that it would probably take him a little while to wake up.

Q) And as a consequence of that, did you and he decide or plan to keep the endotracheal tube in until he had been transferred?

A) Yes.

Angelo then asked him to give a recount of his conversation with Dr. Proper regarding keeping Joe intubated, as best as he could recall it. Dr. Wojdylo; "I think it was just before we began closing the abdomen after the bowel was put back together. He mentioned to me that it was a long surgery, and that he was possibly going to remain intubated for a while. I said that's probably a good idea, we'll arrange for an ICU bed, and that's what we did. We had the resident call on out for the intensive unit bed."

Angelo:

Q) What would be the purpose of transferring the patient to surgical intensive care?

A) That would be so that he could be kept under ventilator, and then he will be extubated when he was ready. There would also be more monitoring. He'd be EKG monitored continuously, and he will have a pulse oximeter that measures the amount of oxygen in the blood.

Q) And what is a pulse oximeter?

A) It measures the pulse rate and the level of oxygen in the blood.

Q) Does it have to have blood flow in order to do its measurements or calculations?

A) Yes.

Angelo certainly wasn't going to miss the opportunity to have a second doctor confirm that blood flow was needed to get an oxygen saturation level. Once again reinforcing that the information in Dr. Proper's note was false.

Dr. Wojdylo then testified that at the completion of surgery, he left the OR, changed his clothes and came to the lobby to see me. He said when he left, Joe was still on the OR table, was still intubated, and still on monitors.

Angelo:

Q) when you left there was no indication of any trouble or any abnormality, is that a fair statement?

A) That's correct.

Q) When you went to the main lobby, did you find Mrs. Nucci and some members of her family there?

A) Yes

Q) What did you tell her?

A) I informed her of the results of the surgery, that we had to take out more of his colon due to the pressure, and that we gave him a colostomy as we had discussed ahead of time. Because of the infection we left the skin edges open, the abdominal muscles were closed, but above that was left open, and that we would transfer him to the recovery room and then to the intensive care unit.

Q) By the way, did you tell her she could probably see her husband in about an hour?

A) Probably an hour to two hours.

Q) When you left Linda, where did you go.

A) I went up the stairs to go to the recovery room.

Q) And why did you go to the recovery room?

A) Just to check on him.

Q) And as you were going to recovery, did something happen?

A) Yes. I was stat- paged back to the operating room.

Q) And when you got to the OR, where was Mr. Nucci?

A) He was on the ICU bed.

Q) So he had been transferred?

A) Yes.

Q) And was he intubated, receiving oxygen, and being monitored?

A) Yes.

Q) Was he awake or conscious or moving or showing any signs of being alert?

A) No.

Q) When you walked into the room, did it appear to you that a crisis was in progress?

A) That it had just ended. There were more people in the room, and the crash cart had been brought in.

Q) Did someone communicate any information to you why you had been stat paged?

A) Yes, I spoke initially with Dr. O'Malley, he said the patient had been extubated and then required reintubation.

Q) Did he give you any information as to how long an interval there was between extubation and reintubation?

A) As far as time in minutes, no.

Q) And is it a fact that Dr. O'Malley told you that the patient had been extubated and then reintubated, and that his heart rate had slowed, but he had responded to medications for that, he told you that didn't he doctor?

A) Yes.

Q) Did you get a sense that there was any chance that damage had been done because of oxygen deprivation from the description he gave you?

A) From that description, no.

Q) Did you talk with anyone else at that time?

A) I also talked with Dr. Proper, and he stated he had extubated the patient because he felt it was safer at that time, because he was fighting his tube. Then laryngospasms happened, and he stated that he got the tube in as quickly as he could, and it seemed to happen within a fairly rapid time sequence.

Q) Is it fair to say you had no concern at that time that this man had suffered any kind of damage as a result of the obstruction that had been reported to you?

A) I was concerned about it, but not at that point, putting all the time frame of events it was hard to tell.

Q) If you were concerned about it, then I take it you would have asked either Dr. O'Malley or Dr. Proper how long did this man go without oxygen wouldn't you? Did you ask that question?

A) I did ask how long had things taken to occur, and I really couldn't get a good answer as far as what the time frame was.

Q) What did they say?

A) They said he had been reintubated quickly.

Q) Quickly, was that reassuring to you?

A) Yes, but again, I didn't know the exact time frame.

Q) And if they said slow, and they took a long time, you'd be worried wouldn't you?

A) Yes.

Q) Isn't it true, doctor, that you weren't all that concerned at that point, because they told you that he had been reintubated quickly?

A) My concern level was low, yes.

Q) Doctor, when you went down to see Linda the second time, did you convey to her any concern on your part about Joe's condition? Did you tell her that you were worried or concerned about Joe's condition or possible outcome?

A) At that point, no, cause I wasn't sure. I didn't want to alarm her unnecessarily, and I didn't want to give her false information.

Q) And did you essentially tell her that he didn't do so well when they extubated him, and he had been reintubated immediately, and that she could see her husband in about an hour?

A) Yes.

Q) Dr. Hollander testified this morning, did you have anything to do with calling for a neuro consult?

A) Yes, I requested his consultation.

Q) And the reason you called Dr. Hollander was to follow up and see whether in fact he had a brain injury, right?

A) Yes.

Q) Did you form an impression that night that this man had suffered anoxic brain damage?

A) Yes, at some point during the night, yes.

Q) The next morning, were you at bedside with Dr. Meyers? Linda came up to you, do you remember her saying to you, how dare you be so casual yesterday when you came down to talk to me about my husband without telling me that something had happened, do you remember such a conversation?

A) I don't remember exact words, but I remember her being angry the next morning, yes.

Q) Do you remember her being angry because she hadn't been told anything with respect to any serious complications that her husband had undergone?

A) Yes.

Q) Did you tell her in that conversation, in sum or substance, that when you talked to her the day before, on both occasions, you did not know that any serious complications had occurred?

A) At that point, I did not know for sure, yes.

Q) And you told her that, did you not?

A) Yes.

Q) Well, was that true, doctor, when you told her in the second conversation he had been reintubated quickly, and you reassured her she could see her husband in about an hour, at that point was it true that you didn't know there had been a serious complication?

A) At that point, yes, I didn't know that.

Q) Did you, yourself, ever consider that the cause of the anoxic brain damage was the heart, or may have been dysfunction of the heart?

A) There was no evidence that he had had a heart attack or damage that way.

Q) There wasn't any evidence of that early on after this event, isn't that true?

A) That's correct.

Q) And later on, you were aware, I take it, that Dr. Mark Thompson, a cardiologist on staff at Rochester General, did a cardiac evaluation. And he found that there was nothing to implicate the heart as a cause of the anoxia and brain damage resulting to this patient, is that a fair statement?

A) That's correct.

Angelo then asked Dr. Wojdylo whether he had personally taken any steps to determine what had happened. Dr. Wojdylo said that the next morning he reviewed the records, and the chart, and had determined that the brain damage was the result of Joe not breathing. Then Angelo asked him if he had made a determination as to how long Joe had been without oxygen, Dr. Wojdylo stated that he couldn't figure an exact time period from the records, but it was at least six minutes, and it began soon after the extubation.

Mr. Faraci:

Q) Can you tell me if whether or not anyone reported to you that this patient was cyanotic at some point before he was reintubated?

A) I don't remember anybody telling me that, no.

Q) What does cyanotic mean?

A) It means the patient becomes blue-colored, and that's due to lack of oxygen.

Both Mr. Brown and Mr. Fox had only a few questions of Dr. Wojdylo, and it was obvious they didn't want him on the witness stand any longer than he needed to be. All of their questions seemed fairly insignificant, but the one question from Mr. Brown that turned my stomach was when he asked Dr. Wojdylo, " When a patient is extubated in the operating room, there is an advantage that the anesthesiologist is right there to take care of any complications that may develop, is that true? Whereas if the patient had gone to the recovery room and had either extubated himself or been extubated there, the possibility of an anesthesiologist being present immediately on extubation was less, is that true?" I think it was at that point that I realized that I hated him as much as I hated his client. I wanted to scream, "You slimy little bastard, what good did it do my husband to have your misfit client extubate him in the OR?" Knowing what his client had done, and I'm sure he knew, he had the audacity to present such an outrageous question like that. These are the kind of cunning questions an attorney can ask when they feel confident that the jury lacks medical knowledge. Again, I was thankful that at least one member of the jury was a Nurse Practitioner. Unfortunately, she wasn't there long.

During Mr. Faraci's questioning, he often referred to the enlarged copies of various documents from the operating room, which he had posted on easel boards. These documents contained very bold alterations of the time changes to which Angelo referred to during his direct examination of the witnesses. Several times we had noticed the Nurse Practitioner lean forward to examine the documents. She would then fold her arms as she leaned back in her chair, glare at Dr. Proper, and shake her head with a gesture of disgust. One evening she received a very disturbing phone call. I don't know the contents of this phone call, but it was disturbing enough for her to become very upset and report it to Judge Syracuse the next morning. She was excused from her position on the jury.

The next witness was Tammy Jo Higgins, the anesthesia technician who was in the operating room at the time of the event. She along with Debra Fader, had been called to start the room turnover at the completion of the surgery. During the discovery phase of the trial, both sides are required to turn over whatever information they have to allow the other side to review, and to prepare for testimony. Michelle Callan had noticed that when the hospital turned over their list of employees who were present in the OR at the time of the incident, both Tammy Higgins and Debra Fader's names were missing from that list. Their testimony would clearly explain why.

Tammy was sworn in and questioning by Mr. Faraci began.

Q) Back in 1994, did you work for a time with Rochester General as an anesthesia technician?

A) Yes.

Q) How long did you work at Rochester General?

A) Three months.

Q) When did you leave?

A) At the end of August of '94.

Q) Last year, at the time you were subpoenaed, did you receive a letter from our firm explaining to you why we wanted to take your testimony, and asking if you would be willing to call us and discuss with us whatever it was that you saw? Mr. Fox: " Objection your honor. She was an employee of the hospital at that time." Mr. Faraci: She was not!

Once again the attorneys argued. Things started getting loud and heated, and Mr. Brown asked that it be argued outside the presence of the jury. The jury was excused, and the arguments continued for quite some time. Mr. Fox and Mr. Brown argued that she was an employee of Rochester General, and Angelo argued that in 1997 when his office had made contact with her, she was not an employee, and had not been since her termination in 1994. She had suddenly become very important for someone they had terminated, and left off their employee list. When the arguments were settled, the jury was brought back into the courtroom, and Angelo resumed questioning.

Q) When you got my letters, the first call that you made to anyone connected with this case, was that Debra Fader?

A) No.

Q) Was it the hospital?

A) Yes.

Q) Who did you call at the hospital?

A) David Watt.

Q) Who is David Watt?

A) I don't know exactly what his position is there.

Q) Well, how did you know to call David Watt?

Tammy stated that her mother was an employee of a doctor at RGH, and when Tammy received the letter from Angelo, the doctor had told her mother that she should call David Watt. She said she called him because she wasn't sure what her standing was in this case.

Angelo:

Q) Now, as a result of that call, at some point the attorneys for Rochester General in this case began representing you, is that correct?

A) Yes.

Q) They had never represented you before, is that right?

A) Yes.

It was obvious that the hospital had no intention of bringing this witness into the case, until they became aware that Angelo not only knew about her presence in the OR, but also knew of her conversation with Kathy Bellucco-Osborne. It was only through Tammy's conversation with Kathy that we were able to learn about Debra Fader. When Tammy told Debra about the information she had given Kathy just two days after the incident, Debra notified her superiors about it. The hospital was not at all happy to know she had given Kathy as much information as she did, and the fact that she had given up Debra's name was a double blow. Tammy was quickly terminated, and the hospital tried to delete her and Debra from their list of employees, hoping that Angelo was not aware of the conversation that had taken place with Kathy. When their plan backfired and they became aware that Angelo had this information, the hospital had little choice but to represent her as an employee and make an effort to control her testimony. They already had control of Debra Fader, since she was still employed there. We were well aware that the hospital had contacted Tammy, and not vice versa, as Tammy had already disclosed that information to a mutual party. Angelo asked her if she still felt a sense of loyalty to the hospital. Her answer was "Yes." Loyal or not, Angelo would still obtain some of the information that was needed from her, but not without resistance. It was important to our case that Kathy testify and confirm the parts of their conversation that Tammy was no longer willing to offer on her own.

Mr. Faraci then asked her to explain the duties of an anesthesia technician. Tammy stated that she would go into the OR at the completion of a surgery, check the cart where all the supplies are kept, make a list of what was needed, then go to the stock room and bring back the supplies.

Mr. Faraci:

Q) Does room turnover have any meaning for you?

A) Yeah. After every case, the room is turned over and prepared for the next case. All the supplies that have been used are replenished, and there are OR technicians that come in and wash the room down and prepare it for the next case. There are also nurses taking out equipment and bringing new ones in.

Q) Is it true that back in August of 1994, on the date you now know was August 11th, you and Debbie Fader were anesthesia techs, and you had occasion to go into operating room number 4 sometime during the afternoon?

A) Yes.

Q) Is one of the things that the anesthesia techs do is to change the circuits on the anesthesia machine?

A) Yes.

Q) And is it true that whenever you're going to change the circuits, the patient would never be connected to the anesthesia machine?

A) Correct.

Q) Usually, is it the case that whenever you go in to do that kind of room turnover, the patient is being wheeled out of the OR?

A) Yes.

Q) And when you walked in to the room this afternoon, when Mr. Nucci developed a problem, it was the usual hustle and bustle of a room being turned over, is that right?

A) Yes.

Q) When you walked in, where was the bed the patient was laying on?

A) In front of the cart, and to the left.

Q) Now, you spent approximately five minutes at the anesthesia cart making your inventory?

A) Yes.

Q) And then you turned and saw the patient, and you saw his face was blue?

A) Correct.

Q) In the deposition last year, you were asked whether you saw that patient turn blue, and you answered it "yes"?

The objections started flying from both sides. Angelo had ruffled a lot of feathers with the word blue.

That was the last thing they wanted the jury to hear, and Angelo was driving the point home as much as he could.

Mr. Fox: Objection your Honor, there comes a point when the same question really ought not to be asked again and again. The Judge replied, " I know what your objection is, thank you sir. Overruled."

Mr. Faraci turned it on again.

Q) Now, you were there five minutes, you turned to leave to go get the supplies, and you saw that the patient's face was blue, is that correct?

A) Correct.

Q) Was anyone excited? Was anybody working on this patient at that time?

A) There was no unusual excitement.

Q) You know what a code is, correct?

A) Correct.

Q) You know what a crisis is, in terms of a patient that's in OR, is that right?

A) Yes.

Q) You know what an emergency resuscitation is, is that right?

A) Right.

Q) Was there a crisis, was there an emergency resuscitation, was there a code going on when you turned and this patient was blue, as you were leaving the room?

A) No.

Q) You left the room, and where did you go?

Tammy stated that she went to the supply room to get her supplies, and returned in just under five minutes.

Mr. Faraci:

Q) When you walked back into the room, is it true at this point Mr. Nucci was still in the same place and in the same bed?

A) Yes.

Q) And was he still blue?

A) Yes.

Q) And now there was a crisis, and a lot of people working around him, is that true?

A) Yes.

She then stated, it was at that point that Debra Fader went up to her and said "you're a student, c'mon, we've got to get you out of here."

Angelo then asked questions regarding Tammy's presence at the gathering in Chameaux Bay two days later and the conversation that she had with Kathy. She admitted to her conversation with Kathy, and that she had told Kathy how upset she had become over what she had seen. But she wouldn't admit that several days later after returning to work, she had called Kathy on the phone. She asked Kathy not to repeat any of the information she had given her, because the staff at the hospital had now told her to keep what she saw "Hushed." When Angelo asked her about that conversation she replied, "I never said that." There was also other important information that Tammy had suddenly forgotten. Mr. Faraci's plan was to put Kathy on the stand and have her testify to the details of their entire conversations, then put Tammy back on the witness stand and question her about it again. I think it's called refreshing ones memory.

Mr. Faraci concluded his direct examination, and as you might guess, Mr. Brown had plenty of questions for Tammy. He would try to spin her testimony as much as possible. Mr. Brown:

Q) Do you know the name of the patient that you saw in the operating room that day? Do you know for sure it was Mr. Nucci, at this point in time?

A) No.

Q) When you came in the room, where was Dr. Proper?

A) At the head of the patient.

Q) Looking right at the patient, facing the patient?

A) I don't know.

Q) Where was he located, as far as the patient's body was concerned?

A) Right in front of the patient.

Q) Next to the anesthesia machine?

A) Yes.

Q) Do you know what time you came in the room or went out of the room?

A) No.

Q) And there were two nurses standing next to the patient, also with Dr. Proper, correct?

A) Correct.

Q) Now, did you ever say any of those things that Mr. Faraci asked you about saying to somebody that the anesthesiologist was not paying attention in this case?

A) I don't ever recall saying that.

Q) Was the anesthesiologist right there, as a matter of fact, in this case?

A) Yes.

Q) Can you tell us when you first came in the room, what Dr. Proper was doing with regard to the patient at that time?

A) No.

Q) Can you tell us what either of the nurses were doing?

A) No.

Q) And any estimates of time that you were in and out of that room are purely estimates, am I correct?

A) Correct.

Mr. Fox only asked a few questions about Tammy's training regarding patient confidentiality issues, and then focused on the fact that as a technician she had no clinical contact with the patients.

Redirect by Mr. Faraci:

Q) Mr. Brown asked you if you know who the patient was. You knew that when you went into OR number four that afternoon, right?

A) Right.

Q) As a matter of fact, when you were up in the Islands and they were talking about what had happened, it was you that volunteered that you were there at the time, isn't that true? They had no way of knowing what you did that previous Thursday, so you're the one that introduced the information to Kathy and others that you were there when complications occurred to Mr. Nucci, isn't that right?

A) Okay.

Q) Incidentally, if you're at the anesthesia cart, where is the OR bed?

A) Behind me, to my left.

Q) But if Mr. Nucci is on the floor bed, then he's someplace isn't he, he's not where the OR bed is?

A) Correct.

At the conclusion of Tammy's testimony, both defense attorneys objected to the testimony of Kathy Belluco-Osborne. They argued that Judge Syracuse should rule her a hearsay witness and thereby exclude her testimony. Angelo argued that she most definitely was not a hearsay witness. Not only was Tammy, with whom she had had the conversation present in court, but the defense also had the ability to cross- examine her if they chose to dispute what she had to say. Angelo stated that the jury should be allowed to hear her testimony and make their own determination as to the credibility of her statements as well as those of Tammy. After lengthy arguments we received a severe blow when Judge Syracuse did rule Kathy a hearsay witness.

The next morning, April 1st, Mr. Faraci called Debra Fader to the stand. After being sworn in, she stated that she was an anesthesia technician at Rochester General, and had been since 1989. She also testified that she was the anesthesia tech working in the OR with Tammy at the time Joe was in there. She described her duties as a technician, just as Tammy had, checking supplies, making a list, and replacing the supplies.

Mr. Faraci:

Q) When you go into the OR, is it termed a room turnover?

A) Yes.

Q) And what else is going on in the OR during a room turnover while you're working at the anesthesia machine or cart?

A) Usually, there are OR technicians that are cleaning up after the case, and nurses are helping out too, preparing for the next case that has to come into the room.

Q) On August 11th, when Mr. Nucci was in OR four, you and Tammy walked in together, is that correct.

A) Yes.

Q) And is it fair to say there was the usual hustle and bustle of a room turnover when you walked in?

A) Yes.

Q) Now, In your sworn deposition before trial, you said from the time you first walked in until you heard somebody say, "Hey, are we going to reintubate this patient, or what?" that time period, in your estimate was about fifteen minutes, wasn't it?

A) Approximately.

Q) You said you walked into the room went to the anesthesia cart, started making an inventory of what needed replacement, started writing it down, taking about five minutes, left to go get the supplies, were gone about five minutes?

A) Yes.

Q) When you came back you went to the cart and started to restock, and were doing your work for approximately five minutes when you heard somebody say "hey, are we going to reintubate this patient, or what?"

A) Yes.

Q) And when you turned you saw the patient?

A) I saw the top of his head.

Q) Well, you saw the face of the patient, didn't you?

A) Yes, from the side.

Q) And you were only a few feet from this patient, and you saw the patients face, and it was dark blue, isn't that right?

A) It was blue.

Q) Did you say it was dark blue at the time of the deposition?

A) I don't remember.

During her deposition, an attorney present on behalf of Dr. Proper had asked her if she would describe his face as light blue, to which she responded, "I would say it was a dark blue." Angelo read her this statement from the deposition.

Angelo:

Q) Did you make that answer?

A) I must have made that answer.

Q) When you turned, and the patient was dark blue, did he have an endotracheal tube in his mouth?

A) I don't remember.

Q) How far were you from the patient?

A) A couple of feet.

Q) You don't remember if there was a tube in his mouth?

A) No I don't, because I just glanced.

Q) Well, that glance was enough to make you run out of that room, isn't that right?

A) I went to get something from the workroom, yes.

Q) Did you run out of that room? He bellowed at her.

A) Yes, I did.

Q) Did anyone ask you to run out of that room?

A) No.

Q) You ran out of that room on your own, Ms. Fader, you knew there was an emergency and a crisis the minute you took a look at that patient, isn't that true?

A) Yes.

Mr. Faraci was becoming visibly angry at her attempts to change her prior testimony. The coaching of this witness was obvious, and I was becoming very angry with her. I wondered how hard it would be to tell the truth had it been someone she loved in that operating room. I could feel the animosity building inside me, and I hoped that someday she would get the chance to find out how I felt.

Angelo then questioned her on who made the statement, "Hey, are we going to reintubate this patient, or what?" Of coarse she claimed she didn't know, and when Angelo reminded her that it couldn't be the anesthesiologist or he would be asking that question of himself, she stated "I would assume a nurse."

Q) When you turned, do you know where nurse Moore was?

A) I don't know.

Q) Was she at bedside?

A) I don't know.

Q) Do you know where Dr. O'Malley was?

A) No, I don't.

Q) When you turned and saw that the patient was dark blue, and you started to run out of the room, where was everybody?

A) They were around the patient.

Q) Everybody?

A) From what I remember.

Q) Well, are you saying nurse Moore was at bedside?

A) She must have been there... somewhere.

Q) Are you able to tell us if nurse Moore was at bedside?

A) No, I'm not able to tell you that.

Q) You don't remember where anyone was? Was the patient still in the bed?

A) Yes.

Q) That bed was right in front of the hallway doors, wasn't it?

Mr. Brown: Object your Honor, asked and answered.

Angelo: Well I can't recall the answer! The judge overruled and made her answer.

A) I have no idea where the bed is. Angelo again referred to her deposition, page 46, and line 15.

Q) Could he have been on a floor bed?

A) Yes, he could have been.

Q) But in any event, was he right in front of the doorway?

A) From what I remember, yes.

Q) Coming from the hallway?

A) Yes.

Angelo: Were you asked those questions and made those answers?

A) Yes, I misunderstood what you said, I'm sorry.

The only thing she misunderstood was that she couldn't change the testimony of her sworn statement once she was on the witness stand, just because she had been told to. Speaking of which, Mr. Brown was sitting at his table and had now developed some head-nodding syndrome. He was making sure not to make eye contact with her, but was obviously nodding his head yes or no to each question that Angelo presented to her. He had done the same during Tammy's testimony. It appeared their job was to stay focused on him, and answer according to his signal. He would continue to do this with each hospital witness the remainder of the trial. I was hoping the members of the jury were smart enough to notice these sneaky little gestures.

Angelo knew once the defense attorneys had gotten a hold of these girls they would try to distort anything that was said in their pre-trial depositions, and he wasn't about to let that happen. His years of experience were apparent, and he questioned them with reference to their depositions like he was holding the Bible.

Angelo's questioning continued.

Q) Shortly after this event, Tammy let you know that she had met some friends and a relative of the Nucci's and there had been a discussion, and the family wanted to know what happened, is that true?

A) Yes.

Q) And she told you that, right?

A) Yes.

Angelo was once again confirming Tammy's conversation with Kathy, and reinforcing the fact that the hospital knew about the conversation, and had therefore terminated Tammy's employment.

Q) Up to the time that you turned and you knew there was a crisis and ran out of the room, was there any indication of a crisis?

A) I don't remember.

Q) Ms. Fader, you're not suggesting that there may have been a crisis going on and you would have been working at the anesthesia cart and not known about it?

A) I would have known if there was something urgent, yes. And the only time I knew there was something urgent was when I left for the fluid warmer.

Q) Have you observed, at least portions of emergency resuscitations, and have you seen codes called and a response to codes?

A) Yes.

Q) Now, if you're in that room and you're at the anesthesia cart and the patient is very close by you, there isn't any way that an emergency resuscitation could go on without you knowing about it, isn't that a fair statement?

A) Yes, I would know about it.

Q) And the truth is, there was no code, there was no resuscitation, there was no crisis at any time before you turned and saw the patient was blue in the patient's face?

A) No.

Q) You know there wasn't any crisis prior to your turning and seeing his face dark blue and running out of the room, you know that, isn't that true?

A) I guess that would be fair to say.

The next questions were with regard to the monitor screens. She stated they were within a couple of feet of her, but she couldn't say if they were on because she wasn't looking. Angelo then asked her if she could hear any monitors emitting any sounds, and if it were possible, given her position so close to them, if they could have alarmed without her hearing them. Her answer was very disturbing. She said, "Sometimes the anesthesiologist tends to turn it down because there is a lot of stuff going on in the room, and they like to keep them down lower, instead of making all this noise." Mr. Faraci:

Q) Are you saying that there are times that you've seen when the alarms are turned down so as to prevent noise?

A) Yes, so as to not disrupt other things that are going on in the room.

Q) But if the monitor sounds, it means the patient is in trouble, doesn't it?

A) Yes.

Q) Is it your experience that some doctors are interested to find out as soon as possible when a patient is in trouble?

She would never get to answer this question, as the objections came fast and furious from both defense attorneys. Angelo had struck more nerves, but he had clearly gotten his point across.

Cross-examination by Mr. Brown started.

Q) You've given us some time periods here, and let me ask you about that. You said you were in the room five minutes, left five minutes, and came back five minutes, approximately. They were all five-minute things?

A) Those are approximate.

Q) So your five-minute block is, at best, an estimate of the amount of each of those times you were in the room, isn't that true?

A) Yes.

Q) At any time when you were in that room, was Dr. Proper in any other position than the head of that patient?

A) Not that I can remember, no.

Q) Was the bed that the patient was on during the course of each time you were in there in essentially the same position?

A) Yes.

Q) And that position was how close to the anesthesia machine and the red cart, approximately?

A) Within a foot.

Q) Now, when you heard the voice that made you turn, were there people around the patient?

A) Yes.

Q) Are you able to identify any of those people?

A) No. (Oops, wrong answer, Mr. Brown will have to help her)

Q) How about Dr. Proper?

A) I know Dr. Proper was there, yes. (Good girl)

Q) Can you identify any of the other people there?

A) No, I can't.

Again Mr. Fox again only asked a handful of questions related to hospital policies, and then Angelo started his re-direct.

Angelo:

Q) In reference to the fifteen- minute period that you estimated prior to the examination before trial last July, before coming to that deposition you met with Debbie White, a nurse at the attorney's office, and with an attorney, is that correct?

A) Yes.

Q) The purpose of that meeting was to review what you remembered, and I take it you reviewed the timing didn't you?

A) As best as I could.

Q) And when you came in, the question was asked about the time, but you made the answers, and you gave the best estimate and your belief as to what you thought the timing was, isn't that a fact?

A) Yes.

Q) Now, you were asked a question about was Dr. Proper at the head of the bed of the patient every time you saw him, and I think you answered, as far as you knew?

A) Yes.

Q) Let me be clear. You worked five minutes at the anesthesia cart before you left the room?

A) Yes.

Q) In that five minutes, is it true you could not see the bed the patient was on?

A) No, I couldn't.

Q) So in that five minutes, you couldn't see Dr. Proper either, could you?

A) No, I couldn't look right at him, no.

Q) So for five minutes, you don't know where he was, or what he was doing, is that true?

A) I was looking at the cart.

Q) So for five minutes you don't know where he was or what he was doing, is that true!

A) Correct.

Q) Now, you left for five minutes?

A) Yes.

Q) In that five minutes, you don't know where he was, or what he was doing?

A) No, I don't.

Q) You say when you came back you went to the cart again, and started working, and worked for another five minutes?

A) Approximately, yes.

Q) And during that five minutes, he's behind you and the patient is behind you, and you can't see him and you don't know what he's doing, isn't that a fair statement?

A) Okay, yes.

Q) And when you came back in the room, the only person you can identify is Dr. Proper?

A) Yes.

Q) Even though you know all of these other people, and you've known some of them for years haven't you?

A) Right.

I was relieved to see her get off the stand. I was so angry it was making me feel sick. My thoughts kept going back to those words, "Hey, are we going to reintubate this patient, or what!" If somebody in that room had said those words, why wouldn't she admit who it was? There was, however, another person present in the room at the time of the event. His name was Abraham Kalachian. Mr. Kalachian was a doctor from Russia, who was employed as a nurse by Rochester General while he was completing his schooling in preparation for his medical boards here in the United States. His name was on the employee list, yet the hospital claimed they had no information on him or his whereabouts and how to contact him. Not knowing where he was located at the present was believable, but claiming they had no background information on a person that they had employed to engage in medical practices was not. An investigator for Mr. Faraci's firm had spent much time trying to locate Mr. Kalachian. He had even made contact with the Russian Embassy, but without enough information on Mr. Kalachian he was still not successful in locating him. The hospital attorney was yet again contacted for information on him, but declined to help. Through a friend at Rochester General, I was able to find out that Mr. Kalachian's employment by the hospital was "Terminated" in Jan. 1995. One would be left to think that maybe he fell under the Tammy Jo Higgins clause. If someone spoke the truth, they needed to be terminated. Knowing he had witnessed the event, I wondered why the defense attorneys' didn't use him to testify on their behalf, unless of course, they didn't want anyone to hear what he had to say.

The trial moved along, and the next witness was Dr. Carafos. Dr. Carafos was an anesthesiologist at Rochester General who was working as the Coordinator Anesthesiologist on the day of Joe's surgery. Dr. Carafos explained that as the coordinator he was aware that there was an emergency surgery scheduled to take place in operating room 4, when Joe's surgery was completed. He stated that he had gone to operating room 4 to evaluate how much longer the room was going to be occupied. When he got to the door he looked in the window. Linda Moore was at Joe's bedside, and upon seeing Dr. Carafos, she motioned for him to come into the room.

Mr. Faraci:

Q) Where was the bed that the patient was on when you looked in the room?

A) The patient was in his own hospital floor bed, and it was adjacent to the operating room table.

Q) Where is the floor bed when you walk in the door from the hallway? How far is it to get to where the floor bed is located?

A) It's probably six to eight feet from the door.

Q) And now, where is the OR bed? Is it to the right or behind or in front of the floor bed?

A) The OR bed would mostly be at the right of the floor bed, but Linda Moore was right next to the hospital bed, so I can't say for 100 percent certainty where the operating room table was.

Q) By the way, how many doors open up into OR four?

A) Three doors.

Q) And how would you describe how Nurse Moore motioned to you?

A) She used her finger and just basically pointed to me to come in.

Q) Did there come to be any sense of urgency?

A) No.

Q) There had been no code called: is that correct?

A) That is correct.

Dr. Carafos then stated that when he walked into the room it was fairly calm, and he walked immediately to the head of the bed, where Dr. Proper was busy trying to manage the patient's airway. The patient was already intubated, and there was no sense of impending doom or urgency. It was then that he looked at the cardiac monitor and saw that Joe's heart rate was 40 to 45, and Dr. Proper indicated to him that he had to reintubate Joe, and was having trouble palpating a pressure from Joe's neck. Dr. Proper informed him that he had given Joe ephedrine, a commonly used drug in anesthesia used to bring blood pressure and heart rate up. Dr. Carafos further stated that a heart rate of 40 to 45, although lower than normal was called bradycardia, and did not necessarly indicate a cardiac problem, however, without a pulse or blood pressure, the patient would definitely be in cardiac arrest.

Angelo:

Q) Dr. Proper said to you that he had to reintubate, and that he couldn't get a pulse?

A) Correct.

Q) Is it a departure from accepted standards of practice for such a patient coming out of four hour surgery to disconnect the oxygen in OR, and not promptly transfer the patient to recovery?

A) Yes.

Q) Doctor, when you have decided to transfer a patient to recovery, how long does it take to get him there?

A) Four or five seconds.

Q) Would it be a departure or bad practice to ever leave the bedside of that patient in the period of time from the end of the surgery to the time the patient is transferred to recovery or intensive care?

A) Yes.

Angelo then asked him to explain the reasons for staying with the patient. Dr. Carafos stated, " Patients are usually fairly groggy, sometimes their airway is obstructed, and sometimes they vomit." He also stated that, " At times a patient can appear to be awake, and will grab at the tube, but once removed the patient can stop breathing. The cause for this being the tube is a very big stimulus, and evokes a response in the patient because it is stimulating their airway. Once you remove the stimulus, most patients continue breathing on their own, but some will lapse and stop breathing."

Angelo:

Q) Do you have procedures in the event someone obstructs or stops breathing for whatever reason, do you have plans for immediately addressing that.

A) Certainly.

Q) Is it important to do so as rapidly as you could?

A) Yes.

Objections again! Both defense attorneys accused Mr. Faraci of using Dr. Carafos as an expert witness. Mr. Faraci stated that he was questioning this witness for whatever information he knew was pertinent to this patient, and the procedures and the subject of anesthesiology as it relates. Mr. Faraci also reminded them that Dr. Carafos was a colleague of Dr. Proper, an anesthesiologist at Rochester General, and was being represented by Mr. Brown as an adverse witness. Apparently Mr. Brown just didn't like his answers.

The jury was made to leave the room, but Dr. Carafos remained on the stand during the arguments and listened. At one point Mr. Brown stated: "He actually can refuse, if he wants to, to give any opinions in this case." The Judge became furious with Mr. Brown, and said, "Are you instructing him to do that?" Mr. Brown: No, but…. The Judge abruptly interrupted him; "Well you just did that by virtue of making that statement in his presence, you've invited that possibility." Mr. Brown: "He's allowed to know that." Judge

Syracuse: "Well, if he's allowed, he should have been told that previously." Arguments ended, and the jury was brought back in.

Angelo continued:

Q) This chart indicates that CPR started about 1350. Where it talked about cardiac and pulmonary arrest, there is a time, 1345. If you're looking at that record, what does that mean to you, 1345?

A) That means that whoever filled this out took a ballpark guess at whether this patient started having some difficulty.

Q) Took a guess? Why would they have to take a guess if they're there?

A) Because this isn't even in the room until after CPR started.

Q) Did Dr. Proper, in that time period, right after you walked in give the patient any drugs?

A) No, I gave the first medication.

Q) Well, who gave the second?

A) I gave the second.

Q) What was it that you gave?

A) Atropine and epinephrine.

Q) What was Dr. Proper doing while you gave the shots of atropine and epinephrine?

A) He was bagging the patient, and at that time they were putting a board under the patient to start CPR.

Q) Now, if we look at this Clinical Intervention Document, what time is the first atropine given documented on this chart?

A) I know the times have been written over.

Q) The record says 1355. Now CPR starts at 1350, according to the chart, and you say you gave the atropine and epinephrine even before the CPR, right? Correct? If I look at this record, the medications are given five minutes after the beginning of CPR, is that right?

A) That's what the chart says, but that is not what happened.

Q) That's not right, is it?

A) Correct.

Q) When, according to this document, does the CPR end?

A) I don't think it says.

Q) Well, how long was CPR given?

A) Approximately six minutes.

Q) Was the person who gave it male or female?

A) Male.

Q) Was it Linda Moore?

A) She's not a male.

Q) Well, I know that. That's why I'm asking you. You're sure it was not Linda Moore?

A) Yes.

Dr. Carafos stated that it requires a good deal of strength to perform effective chest compressions. When a male is present in the room, a female is never allowed to perform the compressions, and he was positive that Linda Moore had not performed the chest compressions on Joe.

Q) When you walked in the room, do you know how long Dr. Proper had been giving this patient oxygen?

A) No. In fact, I don't know the time of events before I walked in the room at all.

Q) When you walked into the room, you were unable to determine what the patient's oxygen saturation was, is that correct?

A) Correct.

Q) Was the pulse oximeter in place and being utilized?

A) I don't recall seeing it. The pulse oximeter also gives us a digital readout as well as a sound that you hear in certain levels of beeps based on the number that it is generating. I don't recall whether the pulse oximeter was even on the patient.

Q) So if the pulse oximeter is there, you would have been interested in learning what the situation was with reference to his oxygen saturation, would you not?

A) Correct.

Q) But you don't remember any value on the screen, or any normal sounds coming from the pulse oximeter that usually emits when it is in use, is that true?

A) Correct.

Dr. Carafos then stated once again that he was aware that the times and sequences on the records had been changed, as well as the length of time he was present in the room.

Mr. Brown started his cross-examination, but it was brief, as it became clear right from the start that this witness, even though being represented by Mr. Brown, was not about to change his testimony, and he was far too intelligent to be manipulated.

Mr. Brown:

Q) You came in through the door from the hallway, am I right?

A) Yes.

Q) Now, taking it from just a little different point of view, if you had come through the scrub area directly into the operating room, would you have been looking at the bottoms of both of the beds?

A) The foot of both of the beds, yes.

Q) They were side by side as you recall?

A) The only one I can remember is the patient's hospital bed.

Q) You don't remember where the operating room table was?

A) No.

I guess taking things from just a little different point of view didn't change the answers he had already given to Mr. Faraci. Realizing he was going nowhere, Mr. Brown directed his efforts into making excuses for the time changes on the records.

Q) Did the hospital always keep their records in military time?

A) No. There was a transition period when they switched to military.

Q) Do you know when that transition period was? Was it around this time?

A) I have no recollection.

Q) Is it true that from the time you entered the room until you left, Dr. proper was managing the patient's airway?

A) Yes, he was.

Q) I have one other question, When you came in, was it your understanding that the patient was pulseless?

A) He had a heart rate based on the EKG, but he had no pressure based on a palpated pulse.

Q) And is it true that any alarm system on any of those monitors can be shut off as soon as the alarm goes off by pushing one button?

A) Correct.

I didn't know why Mr. Brown would reinforce the fact, that Dr. Proper was unable to address Joe's cardiac problems because he was still too busy trying to oxygenate Joe. That being the case, why would he shut off the alarms instead of calling a code to get help? Mr. Fox's questions addressed the fact that a code was not called.

Mr. Fox:

Q) In the hospital there are times when a code is called on the overhead to get people to come to a particular situation, correct?

A) Correct.

Q) Now, in an operating room where there is an anesthesiologist, a surgeon, and nurses, is it the practice of the hospital and your practice to call the hospital-wide code in the event of an emergency situation?

A) It used to be the practice. I believe the practice has now changed.

Q) Why is that doctor?

A) Most of the people that are needed for resuscitation are usually right there instead of somewhere out in the hospital. That concluded Mr. Fox's questions. I couldn't imagine a hospital that doesn't practice calling codes because most people are "usually" there. What happens when the one that's needed isn't? What happens when the doctor involved decides he wants to be a hero, and lacks the judgment to call for help, or has something to hide, such as Joe's case. I also wondered how much impact the lack of calling a code for Joe had on their changing of this protocol. Once again, don't reinforce the protocol to protect the patient. Change the protocol to excuse the doctors failure to adhere.

Angelo started re-direct.

Q) Doctor, regarding military time, any changeover or use, would that affect the minute numbers of time?

A) No.

Q) So any changes on the critical intervention flow sheet that have been written over would have nothing to do with military time, would it?

A) No.

Q) Now with respect to calling a code, when you walked in Dr. Proper was actively engaged in pushing oxygen and air into this man's lungs, right?

A) Oxygen only.

Q) And then you walked in, and you started to address the obvious cardiac problems, and you performed valuable services thereafter, and throughout that resuscitation, correct?

A) Correct.

Q) Now you were there quite by coincidence, and if you hadn't
looked in the window, you probably wouldn't have been there during the resuscitation, would you?

A) It's hard to speculate.

Q) What other reasons would have brought you to the window
or into that OR room?

A) If someone had asked for help.

Q) Right! So unless a code is called they wouldn't have had the
benefits of your help during that resuscitation, isn't that true.

A) Correct.

The next two witnesses were Dr. O'Malley, and Linda Moore. Both
were very reluctant to answer the questions presented by Mr. Faraci.

Dr. O'Malley stated that he was now in private practice at
Highland Hospital. Apparently he was experiencing memory
deficits, as he couldn't recall the answers to most of the questions
he was asked. He did however recall that he was next to Joe's bed
at all times, and not off in the corner of the room documenting in
the chart, as Dr. Proper had stated he was doing during his deposition. Dr. O'Malley also claimed that although he was right at Joe's
bedside, he didn't actually see Joe being extubated, nor did he
observe Joe making any signs that he was ready to be, but he knew
that Joe had been extubated for "some time" before Dr. Proper
made the decision to reintubate him. He also remembered documenting that Joe's condition was not likely a primary cardiac event,
but couldn't elaborate as to why he documented a possible global
hypoxic episode had taken place. He remembered speaking to Dr.
Wojdylo, but he couldn't recall what he had told him. His demeanor
was arrogant and defensive. Much like his documentation in Joe's
chart, he was as evasive as I expected him to be. Why should he
remember such a minor event, it was only one man's life, and certainly couldn't pale to the value of his career.

As for Linda Moore, she displayed a very selective memory of
the event. She too claimed she had never left the side of Joe's bed,

and although Dr. Proper was in her view at all times, she didn't see him remove the tube from Joe, so she really wasn't sure when he was extubated. She stated that it wasn't until she saw Dr. Proper trying to give Joe oxygen with the mask that she realized there was a problem. She also stated that she was not authorized to push the emergency wall button to call a code unless she was instructed to do so by the anesthesiologist, which she had not been. Later she stated that she did in fact have the ability to summon for help. When asked why she didn't, she said "We had all the help that we needed," but then she said when Irene Olds, another nurse who was out of the room at the time, just happened to walk back in the room, she immediately sent her to get the crash cart. She also summoned the help of Dr. Carafos when he too had just happened by the room. When questioned whether a "Room turnover" was in progress at the time of the event, she stated that one was just starting. When Angelo asked her when she had completed her documentation of Joe's condition after the surgery, she claimed she couldn't remember. He brought to her attention that unless it had been done after Joe was extubated, and before he was reintubated, four out of the five boxes that she had checked on the postoperative flow sheet would have been incorrect, clearly proving that she was busy with her charting after Joe was extubated, and not just standing there at the bedside watching Joe and Dr. Proper as she had claimed. She also stated that it was she who started the chest compressions on Joe.

Then Angelo asked her who had altered the times that were changed on the postoperative flow sheet. She admitted that it was she who had written over the original times on the sheet but stated that she didn't know why. She chuckled nervously, and blamed her poor handwriting skills as the possible reason. Angelo then reminded her that handwriting skills were not an issue, as it was only the numbers that were written over.

Angelo's voice had now taken on a very firm tone, unlike his mild manner when he had first started questioning her. She was becoming flustered, and her discomfort was obvious. It was then that Angelo questioned her about the details of the time changes. Angelo asked, "What is the number under the 4 that has been written over?" After spending quite some time trying to avoid answering this question, she obviously realized that Angelo wasn't going to let it go. Reluctantly, she admitted that the numbers under the 4 in the 1345s' that had been written over, were originally 3s'.

That was the answer that clearly exposed the truth. CPR was documented as starting at 1350. If the record revealed that Joe's breathing tube was removed at 1335, which in fact it had been, then the record would reflect a clear 15-minute lapse from the time Dr. Proper removed his breathing tube to the time CPR began. There was no possible way they could explain why there had been no intervention initiated in those fifteen minutes without having to admit that they weren't monitoring Joe and never noticed he wasn't breathing. With the breathing tube removal documented at 1345, it narrowed the gap of time to a five-minute window to which Dr. Proper could convincingly claim that he had spent responding to Joe. Dr. Carafos's sudden presence in the operating room had prevented them from altering the time that CPR began; therefore they could only change the already documented time of the extubation from 1335 to 1345.

Dr. Proper knew Joe's brain was severely damaged long before they started CPR, so he silenced the alarms, and failed to call for help. He didn't want anyone outside of that room to know what had happened. Obviously fear of exposure became his biggest concern.

The witnesses continued to take the stand. Dr. Myers testified that he was not made aware of Joe's condition until the next morning, at which time he was completely shocked and terribly upset. He said he had spent long hours reviewing the chart, and had even spent time on his days off to do so. He stated he was never able to find the answer to how long Joe was without oxygen. He said he had tried several times to locate time intervals that would give him this answer, but his efforts were unsuccessful.

Mr. Brown decided to play in the same mud puddle as Mr. Fox had. He tried very hard to portray Joe as someone who's heart was a bomb ready to explode, but Dr. Myers stood firm, and he stated several times that Joe had no history of coronary heart disease, and that he found no evidence that heart disease caused this problem. He also explained that Joe had experienced many life-threatening complications during his stay at the hospital, and that the last evaluation of his heart showed he still had good cardiac function. Dr. Myers stated, "At no time during his hospitalization did he show evidence of any heart failure, or myocardial infarction, his heart actually looked very normal."

The next witness would support Dr. Myer's testimony. Dr. Thompson was the Cardiologist on staff at Rochester General, who had evaluated Joe's heart after the event. Dr. Thompson's final report stated: "No cardiac abnormalities that could explain this patient's current status." His full report of course was much more detailed. He had documented that Joe's heart had normal muscle contraction, and showed nothing to impair its ability to pump and to circulate blood. He also stated that there were no blood clots in the heart that could have dislodged and blocked a vessel to the brain, causing a stroke. Joe's heart had played no part in contributing to his anoxia, but the anoxia did in fact contribute to his heart failing. He concluded his testimony with the same statement made by all of the other doctors, "The duration of the event is very unclear."

Dr. Grunspan then testified to Joe's overall general health prior to his hospital admission. He stated that Joe had been overweight, but had made great strides in losing the weight over the past year prior to his hospital admission. In reviewing Joe's record, he had discovered that in 1991 Joe had experienced an episode of chest pain that didn't appear to be caused by his heart, but because of Joe being overweight at that time, he referred him to the hospital for a cardiac work-up. That hospital admission was also followed by a formal stress test performed by a Cardiologist, and the results showed his heart was normal. Joe's condition of diverticulosis was discovered during a routine physical. He characterized Joe as doing fairly well. Dr. Grunspan further testified that upon return from his vacation, he had spoken to both Dr. Myers and Dr. Wojdylo. He wanted to see what they knew with regards to Joe's condition. He then reviewed the anesthesia and operative records to try to make sense of what happened during that time. Dr. Grunspan said, "The timing of the event itself wasn't very clear, nor is it clear to me exactly what happened to cause him to be hypoxic." It was Dr.

Grunspan who had requested the consultation with Dr. Thompson, because in his words, "I wanted to know if Joe possibly had a cardiac contribution to contribute to this event." He also wanted to know if Joe could have thrown a clot from his heart that might have caused a diffuse stroke. The test results showed there was no damage to the heart, nor was there any source of a clot that could have arisen from there. Dr. Grunspan stated, "My feeling was he had suffered a primary lack of oxygen first, and the heart was secondary."

Mr. Faraci:

Q) From all the information that came to you, have you formed an opinion as to whether the anoxic event that occurred caused any heart damage to this patient?

A) No, it did not cause any heart damage.

Q) Have you formed an opinion as to how much time, at minimum, this patient was deprived of oxygen in order to have sustained the severe brain damage he did?

A) Not being able to determine that from the record, I suspect it was at least five minutes.

Not being able to determine anything from the record was exactly what the hospital was counting on. They weren't so sure this would be the case when Dr. Dombovy reviewed the records; she was an expert in brain injury. They found an answer to this problem. When Dr. Dombovy received Joe's medical records upon his transfer to St. Mary's, she found that the section of the record at the time the event took place was missing. Someone at Rochester General made sure those records did not come into her possession. Dr. Dombovy's admission note read as follows: "Examination of patient yesterday p.m. and again this a.m., and spoke with family to obtain additional information. Reviewed records this morning. Some are missing from right around the time of the anoxia."

That was the reason she had asked me who Dr. Proper was. She had never heard of him prior to his phone call to her during Joe's admission at St. Mary's.

Omitting information to hide their mistakes seemed to be a real pattern with Rochester General. It was apparent that their staff was trained in this art as well.

Several more nurses would take the stand. All had been in and out of the operating room during the resuscitation or around that time frame. Every question that Angelo asked of them was answered the same: "I don't remember," or "I don't recall." Mr. Brown asked each of them the same two questions: "Where was Dr. Proper when you went into the room?" and "At any time did you see Dr. Proper leave the head of this patients bed?" How could they see him leave the head of the bed? At the time each had entered the operating room Dr. Proper was actively engaged in giving Joe oxygen. The damage had been done long before that. Their robotic answers were very obvious, and very irritating. Angelo asked one nurse twenty-five questions to which he received twenty-five times, "I don't remember." As Angelo turned to walk away from her, the nurse blurted out "Dr. Proper never left the head of the bed!" Angelo stopped dead in his tracks, and he did a head spin that I thought would snap his neck. The anger in his voice was very apparent, as he bellowed, "I didn't ask you that! Is that what you were told to say? Her stupidity was so obvious it created chuckles throughout the courtroom. I personally didn't find her lack of intelligence amusing.

The last witness Mr. Faraci would question before calling on Dr. Proper, was an expert in anesthesiology. Before a medical malpractice lawsuit can proceed, the lawyer must produce an independent expert to support the plaintiff's claim of neglect. Angelo had given Joe's medical records, as well as the witnesses sworn depositions before trial to three experts for review. Two of these experts were anesthesiologists, and one was a cardiologist. All three had not only supported our claim of negligence, but were also willing to testify in court on behalf of that claim. To obtain an opinion from an independent expert, they must be compensated for the time they spend reviewing your case, whether they support your claim or not. If they come to testify in court, there are further expenses to cover their time away from their current positions, travel, and lodging. This can be quite costly. Angelo had chosen just one of the three experts. His name was Dr. Lloyd Saberski. Dr. Saberski was a practicing anesthesiologist and a professor at Yale University School of Medicine. Mr. Faraci opened his questioning by identifying Dr. Saberski's credentials, and the fact that Dr. Saberski had incorporated the review of Joe's medical records, as well as twelve of the depositions given before trial in forming his opinion as to what had happened. Dr. Saberski provided valuable information to explain Joe's condition.

Angelo's first questions were with regard to Dr. Proper's assessment of Joe prior to the surgery. Dr. Saberski stated that although after Dr. Proper's examination of Joe he had documented "work-up within normal limits" he must have had some concerns because of the method he had chosen to put the airway tube into Joe at the start of the surgery. The method he chose was called "rapid sequence induction." He further explained that this technique was not routinely used, but was a very special technique used only in cases where there are special concerns for the patient. This method prevents a patient from regurgitating stomach content, food or acids, up into their mouth during the introduction of the breathing tube.

Angelo then moved on to the drugs that were administered to Joe during surgery, and their effects on the human body. Joe had received both Nurcuron, a muscle relaxant that paralyzes the muscles, and Forane, a gas used to put a patient to sleep. Forane also affects the central nervous system, and sedates brain function. Both of these drugs had been administered to Joe for over four hours, right up to 1:15 pm. Joe had also received a reversal agent called neostigmine to reverse the effects of the Nurcuron. There is no reversal agent for Forane, except breathing, and to force it out of ones system with the administration of 100% oxygen. Dr Saberski stated that Joe was still very sedated when his breathing tube was removed, and he gave a very clear and fundamental explanation why.

Dr. Saberski said, "Forane doesn't just leave you, the problem with these types of agents are that they have an affinity to fat. Forane binds to fat, and if this patient is large or has a lot of fat tissue, even though we may have taken it out of the lungs, he still contains a lot of this Forane chemical inside his body. What you want to do is to replace as many of those Forane molecules as you can with oxygen molecules. You do this by pushing oxygen into the lungs, and even then the lungs may be cleared out, but Forane is still coming back from the various places that it has accumulated in over the last four hours. If the heart is still beating, the circulating blood drives the Forane out of the fat, and brings it back to the lungs. So whereas at the moment just before you stopped moving the air back and forth, there may have been very little Forane in the lungs, but as the blood is coming back from its trip around the body, it starts dumping the Forane back in the lungs. All of a sudden, the Forane concentration is getting higher and higher. If a person stops breathing the Forane can't get out, and starts circulating back into the body. The problem is that the first chunk of blood coming from the heart goes to the brain. The brain is considered to be important, and it gets its share first. As a matter of fact, it's getting the Forane that's been distributed throughout the whole body, it's getting a lot higher concentration of it."

Mr. Faraci Q) What's important about that?

A) Well, the patient will fall back asleep.

Q) Does a trained anesthesiologist know this?

A) Oh, sure.

Mr. Faraci then asked him to explain a pulse oximeter, and the benefits of its use. Dr. Saberski explained, "It is a device that gives you a reading of how much oxygen is in the blood with virtually every beat of the heart." He referred to it as an "early warning system." "If something changes, you know within a second that there is a problem." He further described it as having two alarm systems, one that detects oxygen, and one that detects the heart rate. He explained that if the patients oxygen level starts to decrease, the monitor will alarm with different frequencies to each drop in number. This alarm is designed to give the caregiver sufficient time to recognize a problem, and identify a plan of intervention before the patient is in serious trouble. When in place, this monitor doesn't just suddenly stop." The monitor is designed to allow early intervention. He explained that early intervention was the key to prevent a patient from having a serious outcome. "If you know within a few seconds you're having a problem, you've got a lot of time to figure it out, and to prevent the person from having a serious problem. But if you wait five minutes until they have a problem, you may be wrapped up in a cascade of events, a domino effect, that one system fails after another. The key is rapid response." He also testified that there was no doubt that the lack of oxygen caused Joe's heart to malfunction. "There is no evidence in the chart that the heart had any primary events. EMD is almost by definition an indirect phenomena that takes place to the heart."

Mr. Faraci:

Q) If Dr. Proper observed the patient having trouble breathing, and reintubated him within two to three minutes, in your opinion, would this man have brain damage from that set of circumstances?

A) No, there would be no problem whatsoever. "We know you can start getting irreversible damage some time after five minutes. You've got to make all your decisions lickety-split, and one decision if you can't ventilate is to cut the throat. We're trained to cut into the trachea, because all you've got is time. The only thing that can happen if you wait is a bad thing."

Angelo then stated that two anesthesia technicians saw Joe prior to his reintubation, and said that he was blue. He asked Dr. Saberski if the color blue was significant to the amount of time Joe was without oxygen. Dr. Saberski then explained that it takes time, at least five minutes of oxygen deprivation to turn blue. "Blue is a scientific concept. You have to have a certain amount of hemoglobin that does not have oxygen to be blue. Each time the blood circulates through the body it looses a little more oxygen. When the blood gets back to the lungs it is suppose to pick up more oxygen. If there is no oxygen in the lungs, the blood then starts to lose its red color and turns blue. Eventually all the blood is blue, therefore giving the patient a blue color." Mr. Faraci then ended his questioning by asking Dr. Saberski if after reviewing all of the records and depositions he had formed an opinion with reasonable medical certainty whether or not there were any departures from accepted standards of care on the part of Dr. Proper during Joe's care. Dr. Saberski answered, "Absolutely. The patient was allowed to become cyanotic (blue), which means that at least five minutes had elapsed before intervention was instituted. Also, while the patient remained in the operating room for that period of time to become cyanotic, the patient wasn't adequately monitored to indicate to the physicians and the staff that there was a problem. If a patient has to stay in the recovery room bed for more than five minutes, you have to implement an appropriate safety technique, which is monitoring and giving oxygen. He also stated that if these departures had not occurred, there would have been no problems.

Dr. Saberski's explanation provided scientific proof that Joe's heart was beating long after he was deprived of oxygen. If it wasn't, he could not have turned blue.

It was now Mr. Brown's turn to question Dr. Saberski, and as one might suspect the first questions out of his mouth was how much the doctor was paid to testify. Of course he wanted the jury to believe that Dr. Saberski was not paid for his review of the chart, or his time and travel, but was instead paid to say the things he had testified to. Mr. Brown then spent a great deal of time questioning him on why he did not come to court equipped with the records that he had reviewed in order to form his opinion. Dr. Saberski replied that he had to travel via airplane, and did not feel it necessary to carry all of those records with him on the plane. I didn't know where Mr. Brown was going with this, but it seemed he was doing a lot of spinning in place, and he was being quite nasty about it as well. Mr. Brown then asked him if he could recall anything about Dr. Proper's qualifications, specifically where he had been trained. I chuckled when Dr. Saberski replied, "When I read, I only assimilate the facts that I find useful." With that, Mr. Brown moved on to the fact that Dr. Saberski acknowledged that Debra Fader saw Joe blue.

Mr. Brown:

Q) Do you know what training Debra Fader had in determining the degree of blueness or what that represented?

A) I don't think determination of color requires special training.

Mr. Brown repeated this line of questioning for quite some time, trying to give it one twist or another. He claimed that none of the medically trained persons in the room had documented seeing Joe blue. My thought was maybe they just couldn't decide which one of the time changes they should write that next to. Mr.Brown continued his questioning.

Q) As a trained anesthesiologist, at some point in time you must make the determination that the patient is ready for extubation. It's a judgement call you make, correct?

A) It's a very well educated judgement call.

Q) All right. So you weren't there, but this anesthesiologist made the determination that this patient could be extubated, true?

A) Yes.

Q) And you don't want a patient who has just had abdominal surgery to be bucking on a tube or coughing on a tube, do you?

A) No.

Q) Because that can disrupt the abdominal surgery that was just done, so when you're looking at a patient and you're making all these decisions, you have to keep in mind the type of surgery the patient had, right?

A) Yes.

Q) And so you balance it and you make a judgement call, true?

A) Oh, yes. But there are other options.

Q) Sure there are other options, but that's a judgement call you make every day, right?

A) In this particular case, I think there are other options that might have been worthy to consider.

Q) Now, is it your position in this case that from the time of extubation until the point of reintubation this patient suffered a significant hypoxic event?

A) Absolutely. I think the period of time was much longer than Dr. Proper has stated, based on the fact that the patient turned blue. You need time to turn blue.

Q) Well, actually, heavy people can turn ruddy and blue very easily, can they not?

A) No, I don't think so. There's a difference between being ruddy from venous distention and being blue and cyanotic.

Q) Have you seen any studies on how long it takes for a patient under different circumstances to become significantly hypoxic once oxygen has shut off?

A) Yes, I have.

Given that answer, Mr. Brown apparently didn't care to pursue any further questions on the subject. I was again beginning to get confused. It appeared that Mr. Brown was now acknowledging the fact that Joe was blue, but was arguing how long it took him to get blue. Mr. Brown then stooped to a very childish level in his effort to discredit the doctor. At one point Dr. Saberski had misstated the time on the record that Joe was supposedly extubated. Mr. Brown: "You have your times wrong, Doctor. Do you want to discuss the times? Let's talk about the times for a minute. When do you think that this patient was extubated? When does the record say he was extubated, please?

Mr. Faraci finally bellowed: "Well, hand him the record!"

Mr. Brown: You reviewed it, right? You're here testifying in this Important Case! You should know that. That's something you should know.

Mr. Faraci: "I object to this!"

Judge Syracuse: "That's uncalled for. Everyone who's up here is entitled to a record, and he's entitled to it. Let him look at it." Mr. Brown, holding the record like a child protecting his toy, "I can test his memory, can I not?"

The Judge, "No, not without the benefit of a review."

I was appalled. Mr. Brown stood there appearing proud, like he had just accomplished something significant. From where I sat, the only thing he had accomplished was showing how desperate this defense really was. The same could be said for Mr. Fox. His entire focus was portraying Dr. Saberski as a witness for hire. Then he too questioned the ability of Tammy Jo and Debra Fader to identify that Joe was blue in color. Dr. Saberski stated, "Those are the only two people who spontaneously offered that information." Of course, they were the only two people in that operating room who were not responsible for Joe's life.

It was now time for Dr. Proper to testify. I wanted to see Angelo tear him apart on the witness stand, and he didn't let me down. Angelo started in slow, and discussed Dr. Proper's affiliation with the hospital. He established that Dr. Proper did not have his own private practice, and that all of the patients he took care of were assigned to him by the hospital. Angelo also established the fact that there were no choices of anesthesiologists offered to us. Dr. Proper had been assigned to Joe by the hospital, and had announced himself as "The anesthesiologist who would be taking care of Joe during his surgery." It was clear that he was working as an agent of the hospital. Dr. Proper conceded.

Mr. Faraci then questioned him regarding his assessment of Joe prior to surgery. Dr. Proper stated that his examination had taken place in Joe's hospital room, about 4 p.m. in the afternoon, on August 10th. I had not been made aware of this, and I wondered why it had been done before we had even consented to the surgery. I hadn't met with Dr. Wojdylo until after 5:30 p.m. that same day. However, the assessment was documented, and had in fact been completed by Dr. Proper. He had physically examined Joe, and had also reviewed Joe's medical history in his chart. He had document-ed that although Joe did have some risk factors, they were relative-ly low. I guess that destroyed the defense's theory that Joe was some big fat man with a heart that was ready to explode, and it came from the mouth of their own star witness. Even had that been the case, Dr. Proper was responsible for assessing Joe's risk factors, and addressing them accordingly. That's the point of the assess-ment.

Angelo then moved along to the conditions in the operating room, and questioned Dr. Proper if a room turnover was in progress while Joe was still in the operating- room. Dr. Proper denied that one had even been started. He claimed that he would have put a stop to it if one had been attempted, because it was a deviation from accepted medical practice. This was a man who had just sat and lis-tened as three witnesses before him, including Linda Moore, had testified that one was in fact in progress. Tammy and Debra would not have been present in the room if one was not in progress.

Mr. Faraci:

Q) When you finished surgery and when you transferred him to the floor bed, there was no indication of any problem, was there?

A) There was no indication of any problem when we transferred him, no.

Q) He was satisfactory in every respect, wasn't he?

A) Yes.

Q) Is there any way that such a patient, from two minutes dura-tion of non-breathing, should wind up with severe brain damage?

A) From two minutes of non-breathing?

Dr. Proper had testified in his pre-trial deposition that he had reinserted Joe's breathing tube within two minutes of his extubation.

Q) Well, that's what you said it took, how long did it take you?

A) It took me approximately two minutes or so to get the breathing tube back in, from the time I extubated.

Q) And you could see the obstruction was eliminated?

A) Yes.

Q) This man wouldn't get the severe brain damage that he did get, from two minutes or two and a half minutes, or even three minutes of oxygen deprivation, would he?

A) No.

Q) Is it true that once you eliminated the obstruction he was breathing adequately?

A) I was ——I was breathing for him, but we were ——-we were ventilating him adequately, correct.

Q) Is it true that at that point you reconnected the EKG monitor?

A) When we moved him over he was starting to move. I'm not sure——I don't believe we completed reconnecting the EKG monitor before he was extubated.

Q) Well, isn't it true that you noticed the bradycardia right after you reconnected the monitors?

A) I mean, I first noticed——the first indication that there was a ——-that there was a potential problem was when the EKG, - - - the pulse oximeter monitor, was showing signs of the saturation increasing, and then it stopped picking up, and that was my first indication that there was a problem. And at the same time, virtually, the EKG leads were finished being reconnected.

Dr. Proper appeared extremely nervous. He was squinting and making distorted faces during the entire questioning. He stammered and stuttered through each one of his answers to Angelo's questions.

Mr. Faraci:

Q) Are you saying, Doctor, that you think he was bradycardic before you hooked up the EKG leads?

A) I had——-it was——-.

Q) Did you know he was bradycardic before you hooked up the EKG leads?

A) No.

Q) And the second that you hooked up the EKG leads, you could see on the EKG monitor that he was bradycardic?

A) Correct.

Q) He was pulseless at that point, is that correct?

A) We were unable—-I wasn't able to feel a pulse.

Q) And you don't know if blood was flowing or not at that point, do you?

A) No.

Q) If blood wasn't flowing, the value you got from the pulse oximeter didn't mean anything, did it?

A) The pulse oximeter stopped working, so you're correct.

Q) You said you were getting a value from the pulse oximeter at the time. What was the value?

A) It was into —-into the low 80's or when it stopped working.

Q) That's abnormal isn't it?

A) That's abnormal, correct.

Q) Did you hear an alarm?

A) Did I hear an alarm?

Q) Well, did the pulse oximeter emit an alarm at some point?

A) Emitted an alarm during—-prior to reintubation, there was an alarm, it was on, it was functioning.

Q) It's your testimony that you heard an alarm from the pulse oximeter?

A) I heard—-I don't specifically remember hearing an alarm, but my usual practice is to —-if I do hear an alarm, and I know that it is low, I hit—-there's a pause button on the saturation monitor that I normally hit, because the alarm is loud and disturbing to everybody, especially when you're trying to do things. So I usually silence that alarm, to keep things as quiet as possible.

Q) You heard each one testify no one heard an alarm in that room?

A) I mean, thcy testified—-I think they testified they don't remember hearing an alarm, which I can't comment——I can't comment on that.

Q) But you heard an alarm?

A) I vaguely —-I remember hearing an alarm.

Q) You said "vaguely" heard?

A) I vaguely – I – things were happening quickly. I remember hearing something that alerted me to the fact that the saturation had reached below 90 percent.

Q) You vaguely believe that you heard the pulse oximeter alarm; that's what you're saying?

A) I'm saying something alerted me to the fact that the saturation had gone down below 90 percent.

Q) Doctor, you weren't looking at any pulse oximeter and you didn't hear any pulse oximeter, did you?

A) I was glancing at the pulse oximeter, sure.

Listening to him was far more disturbing than I had ever imagined. The satisfaction of watching him squirm on the stand was hardly worth what I was feeling. I was sick with the thought that this was the person who's hands I had placed my husband's life in. This was just the beginning, and I felt like I was going to explode. All I could do was pray for strength.

Angelo then walked through all the steps that Dr. Proper claimed he had taken to re-establish Joe's airway. Dr. Proper stated that he had put a mask on Joe and tried to break the obstruction by holding positive pressure for about 30 to 45 seconds. (In his deposition before trial, he stated this was done for 45 to 60 seconds.)

When he realized this wasn't working, he then took steps to prepare for reintubation. He paralyzed Joe, and reinserted the breathing tube. Once in, he realized that he had not placed the tube into Joe's trachea. He quickly removed the tube and was easily able to place it into the trachea where it belonged. He again claimed that he successfully re-established breathing within two minutes. At that point, he reconnected the EKG leads, and found Joe's heart rate to be very low, and was unable to feel a pulse.

Mr. Faraci:

Q) At this point, what is your explanation then, for this man having gotten severe brain damage? What happened to this man, in your opinion to have resulted in anoxia that caused damage to the brain?

A) I mean, anoxia of the brain is cause by — um — a lack of supply of oxygen to the brain for a period of — um- - anywhere from three to eight minutes, or somewhere in there. It can come from a couple of reasons. I think that in this situation, what caused the lack of oxygen supply long enough to cause anoxic brain damage was the fact that — um —our chest compressions were not adequate enough to provide the brain with a pulse situation till blood flow, and thereby a supply of oxygen.

There it was, the plan to blame ineffective CPR as the cause of the lack of oxygen and resulting brain damage. This was the reason for claiming that Linda Moore had started the chest compressions. The fact that she is a female would support this claim. It suddenly became clear to me what Abraham Kalachian was doing during this event, and why it was important that he not be made available to testify. They couldn't chance letting him expose that it was he who had performed the chest compressions.

Angelo:

Q) Do you have an opinion as to what caused this heart to dysfunction in such a way that there wasn't any blood flow?

A) There is a variety of causes for what can cause an EMD.

Q) No, do you have an opinion as to what caused in this case, not a variety — but in this case, — EMD?

A) Do I have a specific one possibility that could cause EMD? I don't have one specific one that I can say definitely caused EMD, no. We have a few possibilities.

Q) Doctor, you're aware in this case that the claim has always been that oxygen deprivation, starting with the obstruction, resulted in this man's brain damage, and also resulted in some cardiac failure here. You know that, is that correct?

A) Yes.

Q) And the fact is, any heart being deprived of oxygen can be made to dysfunction in just the way this heart dysfunctioned, isn't that true?

A) That's true.

Q) And oxygen deprivation, because he was unable to breathe, resulted in cardiac problems?

A) That is certainly one possible scenario.

Q) Two or three minutes you took for reintubation couldn't have caused the brain damage, could it?

A) No.

Q) Isn't it true that the two or three minutes of oxygen deprivation couldn't cause this heart to fail in the way it did fail: isn't that
true?

A) That could potentially cause an EMD, absolutely.

Q) Is it your opinion that the two or three minutes that it took
you to reintubate this patient caused something to happen to the
heart, and caused it to fail as it did?

A) That is certainly a possibility.

Q) Possibility! You heard Dr. Thompson, and you know Dr.
Thompson, don't you? He's on staff with a well- known group at
that hospital, isn't he?

A) Yes.

Q) He did the specific evaluation to determine if there was
something about the function of the heart that contributed to the
anoxic event: do you remember him saying so?

A) Yes, I do.

Q) And do you remember him saying that in his opinion, when
he looked at all the evidence pertaining to this heart before, and
during and after, it was his opinion that the heart wasn't involved in
any way in bringing on the anoxia that caused the brain damage?

A) Well, his testimony was that he - - I mean, he looked for any
catastrophic cardiac event that could have caused the EMD. In the
testing that he did, he didn't see any evidence of a heart attack. The
echocardiogram that he did shows there was not a heart attack,
there was no structural abnormality that he could see in the heart,
no blood clots, things like that, so his testimony was that there was
no obvious catastrophe like a heart attack that caused his EMD.

Q) Doctor, didn't he say clearly, not catastrophic, but didn't he
just say that his opinion was that the heart was not implicated in
bringing on the anoxic event? Didn't he say that?

A) He found no evidence of heart attack or structural abnormalities.

Q) No! Did he not state that the heart was not involved in bringing on the anoxic event that caused the brain damage? Didn't he say
that on the stand?

A) I don't remember specifically what his - - what his testimony was.

Angelo stated that Joe had been awake just an hour before, but when delivered to recovery was neurologically unresponsive, well beyond the time of the effects of the anesthesia.

Angelo:

Q) You knew he was in trouble, didn't you?

A) At the time I dropped him off in the recovery room, I did realize that he had anoxic brain damage.

Q) How long was he anoxic? How long was he deprived of oxygen?

A) I mean, the referred - - I mean, how long did the re - - the cardiopulmonary resuscitation go on?

Q) No! Look, he's brain damaged. We know that, don't we?

A) Yes, we do.

Q) And we know that it took at least five and probably more minutes of oxygen deprivation to cause that brain damage, right?

A) Yes.

Q) Now I'm asking you, how long was this man without oxygen? How long was he anoxic and without oxygen, in your opinion? You were there!

A) I mean, I - - the time that I - - that the anoxic event happened was during - - was most likely during CPR. How long did CPR - - in order for me to answer that question, I would need to say how long CPR lasted for.

Q) Well, how long did it last?

A) I have it was - - I don't have a specific time in mind - - a definite time.

It became very obvious why none of the doctors who had questioned him about the event were able to get any clear answers. Confident that even an idiot could see he was lying, Mr. Faraci decided to move on.

Mr. Faraci:

Q) Well, lets not quibble about it. Who did you ask for help during this emergency?

A) Did I specifically ask for - - ask someone to get help? I do not remember.

Q) Didn't you ask Linda Moore, Get help, we need help?

A) Help - - help was gotten very quickly, I do remember.

Q) No, that's not my question. My question is, did you ask

Linda Moore, get help, we need help?

A) I don't remember.

Angelo then read from his sworn deposition before trial. He had stated that he specifically said to Linda Moore "call for help. We need help."

Q) Did you say to her, get help, we need help?

A) As I'm thinking - - sitting here thinking now, I don't remember. I know I said that in my deposition. I don't remember at this point.

Q) At that point, did you need help?

A) Did we need help? Yes, we did.

Q) Did you call a code?

A) We did not. We did not call a code, no.

Q) You could have called a code and gotten immediate response for help, right?

A) We would have called a code if we had needed to call a code.

Q) Well, you needed help, didn't you?

A) We did.

Q) What would it have taken you to call a code?

A) You have to push the button to call a code.

Q) There's a button right there at your station?

A) Yes.

Mr. Faraci reminded Dr. Proper that they only had the benefit of help by Dr. Carafos because he just happened by the operating room at the time that he did to address another issue. He also reminded him that the documentation during the resuscitation was not completed because they had claimed there were not enough people present to document during the event.

At this time Judge Syracuse decided we should recess for the day, and so did I. I had all I could stand of listening to Dr. Proper for one day. In fact, I was so shaken by his testimony all I could do was go home and cry. If a doctor knows he needs help to save a man's life and he doesn't call for it, is that not a reckless disregard for his life? If he neglected him to the point that his life was no longer worth saving, was that not also a reckless disregard for his life? Did having a doctor's license give him the right to harm or kill and get away with it? This was a doctor who had neglected to protect my husband's life, and was willing to neglect him again to cover his own mistakes. He should be spending the rest of his life behind bars, and at the very least, he should never be allowed or trusted to care for another person's life.

CHAPTER X

The night was long, and the ache in my heart was unbearable. I just sat with Joe and held his hand for hours. I couldn't stop thinking how he had reached out for me, and how he had said, "Lin, I'm scared, I'm really scared." I couldn't cope with the pain of the guilt I was feeling for having placed his life in the hands of people with such little regard for it. All I could do was cry and say "I'm sorry Joe, I'm so sorry." There was no sleep for me that night, and the hate was once again starting to control me. My pain was so intense I felt as though my heart was being ripped out of my chest.

The next day Mr. Faraci questioned Dr. Proper regarding the times that Linda Moore had changed on the postoperative record from 1335 to 1345. Dr. Proper denied knowing anything about the changes, or what significance they had. Then Angelo referred to the note that Dr. Proper had written himself.

Mr. Faraci:

Q) Would you turn to your anesthesia record, please? You have a note towards the bottom of it. That note was added on, after this event had occurred, wasn't it?

A) Yes.

Q) And is it fair to say that when you added on this note, the anesthesia record had already been filled out and completed?

A) Yes.

Q) You basically squeezed in this information where you could, and that's the reason why you bordered it?

A) Yes.

Q) And you've got the number 1345?

A) Yes.

Q) What's the number under the 45?

A) I can't say with certainty, but I can't read the number underneath.

Q) Do you remember going back and changing that time?

A) I believe I wrote down the wrong time.

Q) What do you mean by, you wrote down the wrong time?

A) I think I just made a mistake at the time I was writing down.

Q) You wrote the original note, and is it your testimony you changed it right away, right at the same writing?

A) Yes.

Q) You remember that?

A) Yes.

Q) What was the original number you wrote? Was it 1335?

A) I don't know, I can't read underneath there.

I couldn't believe what I was hearing. This man thought the whole world was stupid. I wanted to rip his tongue out so he couldn't talk anymore, and those visions of putting that plastic bag over his head all came back, stronger than ever. Did he really think we should believe that he had changed the time on his own note to match the changed times on the post-operative records? Did he really think we should accept this as a mistake?

Angelo:

Q) When Dr. Wojdylo came up, do you remember discussing whether at that time you were concerned that this patient might have undergone substantial enough oxygen deprivation so that you might be worried that he may have undergone brain damage. Was there any discussion about that?

A) I remember discussing with him that I was concerned with what happened, and I relayed as best I could what happened in the operating room.

Q) Did you entertain the possibility that you might have a brain-damaged person here because of the events that had occurred?

A) It was in the back of my mind, certainly. Um - - is it something that you communicate when you're - - when you're bringing a patient to the - - when I brought Mr. Nucci to the recovery room?

Q) No, when Wojdylo came back. That's before you went to the recovery, isn't it?

A) I did not communicate that concern with him, no.

Q) Did you intentionally keep that concern from Dr. Wojdylo?

A) Absolutely not.

I suddenly developed a clear understanding of why people are scanned for weapons before they're allowed to enter the courtroom. There was now a very fine line between sanity and the rage I was feeling.

Mr. Faraci made several more attempts to elicit the length of time Joe was without oxygen, and Dr. Proper continued to dance around every question that he was asked. Dr. Proper jumped from seconds to minutes, and back to seconds, but ended up with an answer of anywhere from eight to fifteen minutes. Mr. Faraci was becoming so angry with him, I was beginning to think they should have scanned him for a weapon. Dr. Proper continued to blame the EMD and the ineffective CPR for Joe's lack of oxygen, and resulting brain damage. Angelo then reflected to the fact that Joe, by Dr. Proper's own testimony, was successfully reintubated before CPR was started.

Angelo:

Q) Is he getting any oxygen during the time he's being treated with CPR?

A) Yes, he was being ventilated with 100 percent oxygen, yes.

Q) Is he being oxygen deprived totally in that period of time?

A) No. He's getting - - he was getting 100 percent oxygen, and we were doing chest compressions.

Q) Now, before he was reintubated, from the time he obstructed until the time of reintubation, he was deprived of oxygen totally: was he not?

A) Yes.

Dr. Proper then denied seeing Debra Fader in the operating room, even though she had testified she was working at the cart right next to him intermittently for a total of about fifteen minutes.

He also claimed he didn't specifically remember Tammy Higgins testimony when she stated that when she entered the operating room "There was the usual hustle and bustle of a room turnover going on." After Mr. Faraci read back her testimony from the transcript, Dr. Proper then said he "vaguely" remembered her saying that.

Mr. Faraci:

Q) Doctor, if Tammy is correct, and there was a room turnover going on, and if that patient is on the floor bed and still in the operating room, that's a departure from accepted standards of care, isn't it?

A) Yes.

Once again, cross-examination by both defense attorneys was very brief. It then occurred to me that the cross-examinations of all the witnesses, by the defense, had been very brief. It seemed there had been far more objections than there had been questions presented by both Mr. Brown and Mr. Fox. Aside from their attempts to distort the answers of some of the witnesses, and to stop others with objections, they certainly didn't seem to be putting up much of a fight. My first thought was that they just didn't have much to fight with, but Mr. Brown's attitude seemed very inappropriate, and was far too casual for comfort. Something just didn't feel right.

It appeared that Mr. Fox couldn't have cared less what had happened to Joe. His sole mission was to prove that Dr. Proper was not employed by the hospital, therefore they should not be held responsible for his actions. He seemed to be a very cold person, and I simply didn't like him. He was a direct reflection of the hospital that he represented.

Mr. Brown, on the other hand, I found to be very offensive. I felt that he was cunning and sly. When he questioned me, he made a sad face and spoke in a very somber tone. I knew this was to portrait himself to the jury as the very caring and compassionate man that he wasn't, and I found him sickening. Several times I wanted to tell him, "This is a courtroom Mr. Brown, not a theater." If he were representing a client with even a hint of innocence, I could have respected his position. He had the sworn depositions of all these witnesses prior to the trial just as Angelo did, and he knew very well what his client had done. It was he who had encouraged the jury not to decide this case on the basis of emotion, yet it was he who was trying to play the emotion card. He didn't come to court to support any truth, his motive was to distort and cover it. He was living proof that everything does have a price, including a man's soul.

There were only a few witnesses left before Angelo would conclude our case. They were not considered "Fact witnesses," but were there to testify to Joe's condition, and the extensive care he required on a daily basis. Joe's nurses, Veta Nelson and Linda Mohammad would take the stand to confirm that Joe did posses some level of awareness that not just I alone had seen. Our son Nick would explain the various hardships Joe's condition had inflicted on our family. Before these last three witnesses took the stand, court was adjourned for lunch.

CHAPTER XI

With the trial coming near to a close, and the fact that Angelo had proven with each and every witness the sequence of events as they had taken place in the operating room, I knew I should have been able to feel some sense of comfort. He had exposed the facts of why Joe had suffered the degree of brain damage that he did. The evidence was overwhelming and could not honestly be disputed, but I still carried an uneasy feeling that I wasn't able to shake. These were cunning people, but they weren't stupid, and I couldn't help but wonder why they would come to court to fight something they knew they had nothing to fight with. Something just didn't feel right.

We went to a diner about a block away from the courthouse, and after returning from lunch, I was standing outside of the courtroom facing a small hallway where a men's bathroom was located. I watched as Mr. Brown and Dr. Proper exited the bathroom and went back into the courtroom. They were talking and smiling, and seeing this really upset me. I didn't want to walk close to them, so I stayed back for a minute until I knew they were well ahead of me. Much to my surprise, I saw one of the jurors, Mr. James French, exit the same bathroom right behind them. I was of the impression that contact with the jury was forbidden, especially by the attorneys. Furthermore, I wondered what this juror was doing in the hallway. I knew that lunch had been provided for him in the jury room, and he had his own facility to use in the back hall. I didn't know if this was just a chance encounter, but I found it even more disturbing than Mr. Brown's casual attitude.

Court reconvened, and my son Nick was called to the stand. I was trying to stay focused on the trial, but my thoughts were still clouded by what I had seen. I couldn't stop looking at Mr. French. As Nick was testifying, I watched as Mr. French looked at the ceiling and then the floor, and would sometimes glance to the back of the courtroom, but he never once looked at Nick. There was something very suspect about a juror who refused look at the testifying witness. I watched him during Nick's entire testimony, and I knew what I saw, I just didn't know what the significance of it was. At the conclusion of Nick's testimony, Mr. Faraci presented a picture of Joe taken one week prior to his hospitalization. In the picture he was standing next to both of our sons. We wanted to show the jury that he was not the grossly overweight man that the defense had tried to depict him to be. As the jury passed the picture to each other, Mr. French barely glanced at it, and then quickly passed it along.

When Nick was excused from the stand, Mr. Faraci told the Judge that we had concluded our case. The Judge then had an off the record discussion with the attorneys. Then, Judge Syracuse announced that due to the fact that we were approaching Easter weekend, and there was a problem with the availability of some witnesses that were scheduled to testify, court would not reconvene until the following Tuesday. He then stated it would be completed by Wednesday. It was only Wednesday now, and that would mean the trial would be delayed for six days. There was only one day of testimony left, and we could have finished on Thursday and Friday. This trial could have been over before the Easter weekend. Mr. Brown was also claiming that he was now having some abdominal discomfort, and he thought he might require some medical intervention.

I was really furious over this delay, and I found it unacceptable. Mr. Brown was well aware of the time frame of this case. It was his responsibility to have his witnesses available and ready to testify, just as we had. Lack of preparation and a bellyache were not acceptable reasons to delay the trial. This was nothing but a plot to give the jury time to cool down from the damaging testimony they had heard, and God only knew what else they had plans for over the next six days. I also wondered how the jury felt, having to keep their lives on hold for another unnecessary six days. How could the Judge let this happen? How could Angelo let this happen? I was beside myself with anger, and after seeing that little encounter with Mr. French, I was sure they were up to no good. Both of their witnesses not being available and Mr. Brown's back up plan of being ill at the same time was a little bit more than I was willing to accept. This wasn't poor planning on Mr. Brown's part; in fact it was perfect planning. Angelo said it was legal courtesy. Courtesy my ass! This was like calling a time out in a game that you're losing, and they were getting away with it. There was nothing I could do about this except go home and stew in my anger for the next six days.

Court was dismissed, and I left in a huff. As if I wasn't angry enough, Joe's sister Darlene came up to me in the lobby outside of the courtroom. She said "Did you see that juror on the end, that guy French? He wouldn't look at Nick while he was testifying. It was like he went out of his way not to look at him. What was that all about?" I said, "That's a good question, what was that all about? I saw him too, and I don't know what to make of it." I then told her that I had seen him coming out of the men's room right behind Mr. Brown and Dr. Proper, and that I wasn't feeling very good about it. I still didn't know what the significance of it was, but I was glad that others had noticed him as well. Darlene said, "Yeah, we all saw him." Now I was convinced that the delay was planned. I was also convinced that the trial delay and the bathroom encounter were somehow connected. I tried not to let my feelings get the best of me. The evidence was so strong, it would take more than Mr. French to dig them out from under all the testimony the jury had already heard.

CHAPTER XII

Over the next five days I spent most of my time thinking about the testimony of all the witnesses who had taken the stand. Mr. Faraci had concluded our case, and although some witnesses had not been as forthcoming with the truth as others had, I was very satisfied with the information he was able to obtain from each witness. The timing and sequence of events that had taken place in that operating room couldn't have been made any clearer. Dr. Proper's testimony, although upsetting for me, had contained holes that were big enough to drive a truck through. The changing of the times and false information on the records, as well as the time changes on his very own vaguely written note were more than obvious. His refusal to communicate any information to other doctors with any clarity or honesty about what had happened. His admission that he knew Joe had suffered anoxic brain damage, and his failure to communicate that information to Dr. Wojdylo told the story all by itself. His sickening admission that they needed help, and his refusal to call a code to obtain that help. All had been exposed with precision on Angelo's part.

The most important information came from the five doctors who had clearly testified that Joe's heart had failed due to a long period with lack of oxygen, but that the heart itself had played no part in bringing on the anoxic event. After all their testimonies Dr. Proper still tried to claim Joe's heart was the cause of his brain damage. To believe Dr. Proper, you would have to assume that these five doctors, who were very prominent and successful in their fields, and who were actually employees of the hospital, would put their reputations and careers on the line just so they could come to court and testify against him. The testimony of the two anesthesia technicians who had seen that Joe was dark blue before he was reintubated reinforced the doctors' testimonies, and was further proof that Joe was neglected for a very long time before it was noticed that he wasn't breathing. Angelo couldn't have exposed the truth for this jury any better if he had gift-wrapped it. I was confident that this wasn't just my opinion. I had received phone calls from various people who were also present in the court, and had also listened to the testimony. Some of these people were lawyers themselves. All were in agreement that Angelo had done an awesome job uncovering the truth. It was obvious that he had contemplated every possible attempt of manipulation the defense could think of, and was more than ready for them. He had obtained information from every hospital employee as though they were our own witnesses. I was still upset that he let them get away with the delay in the trial. Maybe he couldn't have done anything about it, but I wanted him to at least fight like hell to try and stop them.

CHAPTER XIII

It was now Tuesday morning, April 14th and we returned to court. It appeared that Mr. Brown's bellyache was now okay, and he called his first witness, Dr. John Bennett. Dr. Bennett was the Chief of Cardiology at Albany Memorial Hospital.

Before reviewing his credentials, Mr. Brown was careful to point out that this was Dr. Bennetts' first time on the witness stand in court. I gathered his point was to convince the jury that Dr. Bennett was not a paid witness, but had come to support Dr. Proper out of the goodness of his heart.

Mr. Brown first had Dr. Bennett explain EMD, and it's potential cause and effects. Dr. Bennett testified, that a decrease of blood flow to the heart would initiate EMD, and of course, Dr. Bennett had a much different theory than all of the other doctors as to what had caused this to happen to Joe.

He said, "When someone is trying to exhale against a fixed obstruction in the vocal cords, there is tremendous pressure exerted on the heart. This in turn decreases the blood returning to the chest cavity, so the blood does not come back to the heart, and the heart doesn't fill. The heart then cannot beat, and that is one of the causes of EMD." However, he forgot to mention that if the intervention to the obstruction is quick, the patient never gets to the point of EMD.

Mr. Brown:

Q) In your opinion, under these circumstances, how long would it take a person such as Mr. Nucci to demonstrate blueness on the side of his face?

A) I think that could happen very quickly, certainly within two to three minutes. He's really straining to try and breathe against the obstruction, and that distends the neck veins. These patients will always have a ruddy kind of look to the head. So I think there are a number of reasons why he might have looked blue.

His answer was absolute bullshit. Of course everyone quickly gets ruddy in appearance when they're choking, but nobody ever said they saw Joe choking, or that he looked red. Dr. Saberski had already explained there was a very distinct difference between becoming ruddy looking from venous distention and being cyanotic. Mr. Brown:

Q) And in your opinion, how long a period of time would this patient - - would it take for that to start demonstrating that color change? (He was careful not to say blue)

A) Very, very quickly, I would say just two minutes or so. That's not going to take very long.

Mr. Brown continued questioning Dr. Bennett for quite some time. All of his questions were repetitious with regards to how quickly a patient can turn colors. He finally concluded his questioning with " Doctor, have you formed an opinion, based on your review of this chart, at what point in time this patient suffered anoxic encephalopathy?

A) Yes, I have.

Q) And can you give us the benefit of that opinion?

A) I think the brain was deprived of oxygen for a prolonged period of time, really during the resuscitation. The period of time the patient was hypoxic from the obstruction was quickly turned around, yet the resuscitation was much more prolonged than that. And that is where you really have to look for the time that the brain was oxygen deprived, and the brain was oxygen deprived because the blood was not circulating. It was clearly difficult to effectively resuscitate this man because of his large size and because, you know, he just had an operation, and the effectiveness of CPR really drops in that setting. Mr. Brown, once again practicing for his acting career, chuckled, and jokingly asked the doctor if he intended to charge him for reviewing the records, and for his time away from his practice to come and testify, to which the doctor of course responded, "Yes."

Mr. Faraci:

Q) Doctor, when were you first contacted with respect to this matter?

A) I have to think. I can't give you an exact date.

Q) Well, was it the past couple of months?

A) Yes.

Q) And were you told that the case had already been set down for trial, and were you given a trial date?

A) "I don't think so, I really don't remember."

Q) Other than the depositions and the hospital records, did you receive a summary of this case?

A) You mean like a summary of the case written by a lawyer or somebody?

Q) Well, I mean a summary. Did you get some kind of information saying Joe Nucci was admitted on such and such a date, the admitting diagnosis was such and such, he was treated, an operation occurred, this is what happened, here's what we're looking for, what we'd like you to do. Did you receive anything of that type?

A) Anything written like that, not that I can recall.

Q) When you started your review, did you have any information as to what it was that you were suppose to be looking for or what opinions you were supposed to be at least considering?

A) No.

Was he suggesting that Joe's chart just showed up on his desk one day, and he started reading it?

Q) Now, I take it when you reviewed the depositions and the hospital records, you got a flavor of what the issues were?

A) Oh, yes.

Q) And when you reviewed the chart, did you look to see, for example, what time bradycardia started and what time it ended?

A) That is one of the things we looked for.

Q) Well, what time did it start and what time did it end?

A) Well, that's difficult to get at.

Q) "Why is that?"

Dr. Bennett then spent some time shuffling through several volumes of papers. After getting to the pages he needed, he asked to have the question repeated.

Q) What time did bradycardia start and what time did it end?

A) The bradycardia was noted, according to the note, immediately after he was reintubated.

Q) Well, it was noted immediately after the EKG leads were reconnected, isn't that true?

A) Well, EKG leads would have to be on for them to note the bradycardia.

Q) Didn't you get the sequence that the patient obstructed, he was reintubated, and the EKG leads were reconnected, and bradycardia was noted?

A) Correct.

Q) And then pulselessness was noted immediately thereafter, is that correct?

A) Correct.

Q) How long was the bradycardia? Give us a time as to how long it was in effect.

A) I think it was around 1350 or so, or sometime between 1345 and 1350. It's unclear.

Q) Excuse me, why is it unclear?

A) Because there is a code, and it's very difficult to know minute to minute times.

Q) Doctor, where do you see evidence of a code?

A) The patient was being resuscitated.

Q) Doctor, you have to call a code in order to have a code, don't you?

A) No.

Q) Really?

A) Yes.

Q) What does code mean?

A) You're talking about resuscitating a patient. Everyone was there who was necessary to resuscitate that patient.

Q) You say there was enough people there. Do you know how Dr. Carofos got into that room?

A) He was walking by and walked in.

Q) If Nurse Moore didn't motion to him to come in, he wouldn't have been there, would he?

A) I don't know that.

Q) Well, how else would he get there, unless someone summoned him or unless a code was called?

A) I don't know that, I wasn't there, I can't speak to that.

Q) Oh. Well, then, is it fair to say you don't know if there were enough people in that room at the time of resuscitating the patient, isn't that true?

A) No. Dr. Proper was there, and several nurses.

Q) How do you know there was enough people there to help under the conditions? You weren't there.

A) I wasn't there, but from what I read, there were several people there.

Q) You mean from what you read, was that Dr. Proper said there was enough people there, right?

A) That was one of the pieces of information, yes.

Q) Do you know if there was anyone at the crash cart that was documenting and dispensing supplies? Do you?

A) I wasn't there.

Q) Well, I know you weren't there, but you have come here to give an opinion, and you did base it on the review of the chart and the depositions. Do you recall any information indicating that someone was at the crash cart documenting and dispensing drugs, supplies, whatever was needed during the resuscitation?

A) I don't recall any information on it.

Q) Oh, the doctor doesn't run back to the crash cart, somebody ought to be at the crash cart that's documenting what the doctors are doing, isn't that the procedure?

A) That is often done.

Q) That's always the procedure, isn't that true?

A) That is often - - that is often the procedure in most hospitals.

Q) When did EMD start? What time did it start according to the records that you reviewed? When did this heart stop?

A) This heart stopped sometime after extubation.

Q) Well, can you fix a time?

A) The patient was extubated at 1345, and I think it happened sometime between 1355 and 1350.

Q) Where did you get the 1345 from?

A) It was in the records as the time of extubation.

Q) Well, did you note that many of those times were changed?

A) There were some instances where there was some times changed.

Q) As a matter of fact, 1345 was changed, wasn't it?

Angelo then referred to the court testimony of Linda Moore when she had stated that the 1345 had been changed from 1335. Dr. Bennett: "I don't remember that." Angelo, "Well let me show it to you. Angelo then referred to document 4-D marked in evidence.

Q) "Documentation of care." Do you see that?

A) Yes.

Q) Now, that was changed, wasn't it, to a 1345?

A) Well there is definitely - - Yes. But if you're asking me what I see, all I can tell you is there is clearly a 4 there.

Q) Is there clearly something underneath it?

A) Yes, but I can't tell you - -.

Angelo: "Nurse Moore testified that was a 3."

Objections started once again by Mr. Brown. Quite frankly, I had been wondering what was taking him so long. Mr. Brown: "That's not what she said at all."

Angelo: "Well, lets get it out." Angelo promptly displayed the portion of the record with Nurse Moore's testimony stating that the four was originally a three. Angelo continued drilling Dr. Bennett on the time changes of various records for quite awhile. Dr. Bennett then stated, "Nurses don't always know what to document."

Angelo:

Q) Are you saying the nurses were not well trained?

A) No, I'm not saying that.

Angelo then pointed out that collectively the nurses had over twenty years of operating room experience.

Q) All these experienced people, and we couldn't get accurate documentation according to the procedure that exists at that hospital as to what happened during this resuscitation, it that right?

A) I'm not sure that's right, but it certainly isn't unusual.

Q) Is that how they do it at your hospital, Doctor?

A) What you have to realize is happening is you're trying to save someone's life, and yes there are policies and procedures to write everything down.

Q) The nurse who's at the cart is not trying to save someone's life. Her job is to document, isn't it?

The witness: "Can I interrupt him?"

Judge Syracuse; "No Doctor, answer the question."

Mr. Brown; "Your honor, I object to the interruption. He can always - -

The Judge; " I said he should answer the question."

Mr. Brown: "I thought he was, Your Honor."

Judge Syracuse; "He was making some comments. That's not answering the question."

The situation was starting to get very heated, and the doctor finally stated, "That is one of the things they do, yes."

Angelo: "That wasn't done here, you don't see any specificity as to what happened during the course of this resuscitation, do you?"

A) That's correct.

The doctor was still trying to insist, against the obvious, that Joe's brain damage had occurred during the resuscitation period, and not before. Thank God Angelo had done his homework.

Angelo:

Q) When he starts to fight, and tries to breathe, isn't the first thing that happens is that his heart rate goes up and his blood pressure goes up, not down?"

A) For perhaps a minute or so.

Q) Now in this instance, you don't see any evidence, do you, that there was ever a notation that the blood pressure and the heart rate go up? Isn't that true?

A) Correct.

Q) The first time that they noted anything with reference to this patient was when they reconnected the EKG leads and they noted the heart rate was going down. Now, the increased heart rate and high blood pressure had already occurred, hadn't it?

A) Presumably.

Q) Yes. And, of course, they didn't pick that up because you know that the heart rate and rhythm were not being monitored before that, were they?

A) They were not monitored as they were transferring him to the bed.

Q) He was already on the bed. You yourself said the EMD didn't start for five minutes.

A) Yes, but they transferred him to the bed, as I understand it, and then he developed this tremendous laryngospasm, and their first goal was not to put on the heart monitors, but to reintubate the patient, which they promptly did.

Q) "First goal!" Doctor, he was on the floor bed for a period of time before he obstructed, wasn't he?

A) Correct.

Q) And you know the first move of the heart rate would have been up, not down, right?

A) Very briefly.

Q) Sometimes not so briefly, huh?

A) Sometimes.

Q) Did I understand you to say that it takes two to three minutes to turn blue under these conditions that Mr. Nucci had?

A) No. I said the rate at which someone will get cyanotic depends on a lot of things, not the least of which is the color of the patient's face, you know, that's a very difficult thing.

Q) Well, you had a description here of Debbie Fader indicating that this man's face, when she turned, was dark blue. Remember that?

A) That's what she said.

Q) Do you have any reason to doubt it?

A) No.

Q) Well, if it's dark blue, how long did it take to get dark blue?

A) Well, I think to turn dark blue - - well, to turn blue would be - - I believe what is very important in this case was the high intrathoracic pressure as he strained against his laryngospasm, distending the neck veins, and I think it can all happen fairly quickly, as I said, within, two minutes or so.

Q) Did you read that part of her testimony where she said before she saw the patient, and saw that he was dark blue, someone said quote, "Are we going to reintubate the patient?" end of quote, do you remember reading that?

A) No, I don't.

Q) Well, does that tell you this man had been without oxygen at least two to three minutes before being reintubated? And this was prior to reintubation, if she's correct, isn't that true?

A) If she said that, yeah.

Angelo then moved on to the testimony of Tammy, and the fact that she had also seen that Joe was blue before any measures of intervention were made. Dr. Bennett stated that there was no doubt that Joe had to have been cyanotic at some point, and that in his review he had only relied on the documentation of the medically trained staff.

Angelo then asked him if he found any documentation by the medical staff that Joe was cyanotic at any time, to which he of course had to answer, "No." If there was no doubt that Joe had to have been cyanotic, didn't he find it suspicious that no one had documented that?

Angelo then reminded Dr. Bennett that Dr. Thompson had specifically tested Joe's heart to determine if it was the cause of the anoxia that he had suffered, and he had concluded that it played no part in Joe's condition. Dr. Bennett agreed that it was not the primary cause, but continued to support his theory that it did play some part in the length of time Joe was without oxygen. When Angelo offered the testimony of the other doctors to him regarding their opinions that the heart was not implicated, Dr. Bennett stated that he had not seen any notes with regard to their testimonies.

It would appear that Dr. Bennett had seen only the notes that the defense had wanted him to see. I'm not so sure that he was just an innocent party, but it did seem that he had definitely been sandbagged to a certain degree. Once again, eliminating information seemed to be the overall practice on the part of the defense, even to their own witnesses. When he was finally dismissed from the stand, his demeanor suggested it would probably be a very long time, before he would be willing to testify in court again.

The defense then presented their next expert witness, Dr. Geraci. Dr. Geraci was an anesthesiologist who had once practiced at Genesee Hospital, and was now affiliated with the National Naval Medical Center in Bethesda, Maryland.

Dr. Geraci stated he had testified in court as an expert only one time before this case. Mr. Brown had chosen two first time witnesses, or maybe he didn't have much choice at all. Could it be he was trying to benefit from their inexperience, or was he not able to con anyone who was experienced enough to know how to review a chart in it's entirety, and refused to let themselves be set up. Whatever the case, Dr. Geraci's testimony went pretty much the same as Dr. Bennett's had. He reviewed each step that Dr. Proper had taken during his reintubation of Joe. He stated that he could find no malpractice involved in this case, and Dr. Proper had done everything that could be expected of any reasonable and competent anesthesiologist. He also stated, as Dr. Bennett had, that he believed that Joe had suffered all of his brain damage during the period of time that CPR was being given, and not before.

Mr. Faraci was quick to show that this witness was clearly lacking the facts from the testimony of several witnesses. Dr. Geraci had elicited all of his information from the testimony and sworn statements of only Dr. Proper. He did not recall the testimony of Debra Fader, Linda Moore, Dr. Wojdylo, and many others. He did recall the testimony of Dr. Carafos, but chose to acknowledge that of Dr. Proper's instead. I guess that would be the courteous thing to do, after all, Dr. Proper was the one paying him. He, like the others, could not determine any times of the event. He was very surprised to hear testimony that a room turnover was in progress, and stated "I have never worked anywhere where I've seen that done. I would say it would be most unusual. It's unheard of to turn over a room while the patient is still in the room." He must have briefly forgotten who he was testifying for when he stated that any competent anesthesiologist who was continuously monitoring his patient should be able to detect a problem within seconds, and reintubate within a minute or two at the most, and prevent further complications. Of coarse, he must do this before the patient turns blue.

We had finally come to the very last witness. Mr. Brown called Dr. Proper to the stand to testify on his own behalf. This time Dr. Proper displayed a much different attitude. He appeared to have been well coached, and for some reason had now taken on an air of confidence. Maybe the six-day delay had been very helpful for him, just like the thirty-hour delay before telling me what happened to Joe. In fact, it appeared that he could do everything better after a delay, including responding to his patients. This time he spoke like a bold-faced liar. Mr. Brown asked him to give a narrative account of exactly what happened, according to him.

This was his story:

"I turned the Forane off at 1335, and gave him a medication to reverse the effects of the muscle relaxant that was still in effect. I then placed Mr. Nucci on 100% oxygen. At about 1338, I checked Mr. Nucci for return of function. At about 1339 Mr. Nucci began breathing spontaneously, but still no signs of him awakening. At about 1340 I had the hospital bed brought into the operating room, and the bed was brought in at about 1442. (Oops), I left the pulse oximeter in place, and I did disconnect the oxygen for five or ten seconds. Once he was moved to the bed, I immediately hooked him back up to the oxygen, and the pulse oximeter was in place. At this point he started showing signs of awakening, and began moving his extremities. He was reaching for his tube, and at 1445 I decided to remove the breathing tube. At the first breath he showed signs of obstruction, and I asked him if he was having trouble breathing. He said - - he shook his head yes." He then explained all the steps he had taken to reintubate Joe. " The pulse oximeter had gotten down to about 75 percent, and the heart rate started to climb over the course of the next fifteen or thirty seconds, or so, and got back up into the low 80's, and then all of a sudden it stopped picking up. This was while the reintubation process was going on, and after he was successfully reintubated, the EKG leads had been reconnected, and Mr. Nucci's pulse was approximately 40 to 50. I checked for a pulse, and did not feel one, and that was approximately 1449. I gave a medication called ephedrine, which is a medication that we typically use when someone has low blood pressure. At that point, that's when Dr. Carafos entered the room. Dr. Carafos grabbed the atropine and epinephrine, and gave those, and we - - we- - CPR began at approximately 1350. Mr. Brown then asked Dr. Proper where Linda Moore was, and he answered, " She was to my left, to my left. I'm standing at the head, she was to my left, probably a third of the way down the floor bed." Then Mr. Brown, once again playing the drama king, spoke very softly and said, "You're under oath, you understand that?" Dr. Proper replied, "Yes."

Wow! After four years, what an amazing memory, what an amazing story, even though he had just misstated several of the times, jumping from 13 to 14. I wonder where all of that information was documented. Where had he been hiding all of those detailed minutes of time that so clearly explained what happened? His story was so impressive I couldn't imagine why he hadn't been willing to share it with all those doctors who were desperately trying to figure out what had happened, and how long Joe had been without oxygen. I'll bet he had those times written down at home, or maybe his lawyer was saving that information for him.

It's terrible how all the witnesses had all lied except for him. Why did Tammy and Debra Fader both say that Joe was dark blue before Dr. Proper reintubated him? Maybe no one should believe them anyway, they were only there for the room turnover that Dr. Proper said wasn't happening. Linda Moore must really dislike him. She testified that she was on his right facing the door, and had motioned for Dr. Carafos to come into the room when he appeared in the window. Now Dr. Proper told us, positively, that she was on his left, which clearly puts her back to the door, so she couldn't possibly have seen Dr. Carafos look into the room, let alone motion for him to come in. And wasn't it lucky for Dr. Proper that he suddenly remembered that Joe's heart rate had gone up before it went down. Maybe Angelo reminding Dr. Bennett that that's the way it works jogged his memory. I didn't know how he had figured that out though, the EKG leads weren't reconnected yet, and I thought Dr. Proper had previously testified that the pulse oximeter had stopped working before the EKG leads were reconnected. Dr. Thompson and Dr. Hollander had been especially nasty to him. They had the nerve to say that it was a lack of oxygen that caused Joe's heart to stop, and now, thanks to Dr. Proper, we know the results of all those tests they performed on Joe must have been wrong. I guess it was just a coincidence that the cardiac and the neurological tests had both concluded that the anoxia was caused by lack of oxygen, unrelated to Joe's heart. How could everyone not think that all those time changes on the records were not just simply honest mistakes, after all, Dr. Proper said so. And why wouldn't we think that at 1342 Joe had shown no signs of being awake, but three minutes later, at 1345 he was so awake he needed to have the breathing tube removed, after undergoing this major and lengthy surgery. Of course Dr. Proper had exercised good judgment by removing the tube that early. He didn't want Joe to injure his fresh abdominal incision by fighting against the tube, and simply putting him back to sleep was an option he forgot to entertain. Poor Dr. Proper, being the only one that was telling the truth must have made him feel so isolated. How unlucky for him that even Dr. Dombovy couldn't support his theory, but then again, she didn't have any records from the time the event took place. It was too bad how they had mysteriously been removed from Joe's medical chart before it was sent to her.

To this day, I don't know what stopped me from physically attacking him, and that conscienceless actor that called himself a lawyer.

CHAPTER XIV

Court recessed for the day, and reconvened at 9:30 a.m. on Wednesday. We then heard the closing arguments presented by each attorney.

Mr. Fox was first, and stated that no one who was employed by the hospital had been accused of doing anything wrong. Although the hospital did support Dr. Proper, he definitely was not an employee of Rochester General Hospital, and they were not responsible for his actions. Dr. Saberski must have really gotten under his skin, because he did spend some time making derogatory remarks regarding his being a " Big shot" from Yale.

Mr. Brown once again took center stage, and very emotionally stated that of coarse this was a very sad case, and if Dr. Proper had done anything wrong, he should be held responsible. But, Dr. Proper had done nothing wrong, and he was in no way responsible for what had happened to Joe.

Mr. Faraci's argument was far more detailed than the others. He briefly reviewed the testimony of many of the witnesses, pointing out the numerous contradictions between all of their statements, and those of Dr. Proper. He informed the jury that medical charting is a legal document that comes with standards and requirements, and is not to be altered. "It's not like a personal diary, and you can't just pick and chose if you want to write something or not." People's lives depend on that documentation, and this was something that Dr. Proper was well aware of."

Angelo then told a wonderful story of Susanna, from the Book of Daniel. "Susanna was a beautiful young wife in the days when the Elder Judges would travel around to different districts. Two of them were not men of character, and came across Susanna one day, and approached her when she was alone in her husband's garden. They told her that they were going to have their way with her, and if she refused they would tell everybody they found her engaged in adultery. At that time, adultery was a capital crime. Susanna was of character, and she refused, so the Elders did as they had threatened, and she was convicted. She appeared before young King Daniel, who, they say thirsted for justice, and Daniel said, before I pass sentence, I want to ask these people some questions. He had the Elders brought before him one at a time. He then asked the first Elder what tree he had seen Susanna and the young man under. The Elder answered "The Cedar tree." They then brought in the second Elder, and Daniel asked him what tree he had seen Susanna and the young man under. He answered "The Mastic tree." Daniel knew there was a great deal of distance between the two trees, and he set Susanna free. Thus became the rule of cross- examination, and questioning witnesses one at a time to elicit the truth."

Angelo strongly encouraged them to look for the truth, look for the distance between the trees. He then reminded them that one day either they, or, someone they loved would be hospitalized, or have the need for surgery, and the standards they set with their verdict could make a very big impact on their own level of care.

We broke for lunch, and when we returned the judge gave his instructions to the jury before they would begin deliberating. Judge Syracuse read the instructions from a pre-written set of legal guide-lines. I was appalled at the wording in the instructions, and how clearly they were designed to protect the accused doctor. He read; "The standard to which a doctor is held is measured by the degree of knowledge and ability of the average doctor or anesthesiologist in good standing in the medical community in which the doctor practices. In performing a medical service, the doctor is obligated to use his best judgement and use reasonable care. By undertaking to perform a medical service, a doctor does not guarantee a good result. The fact that there was a bad result of the patient, by itself, does not make the doctor liable. The physician is liable only if he was negligent. Whether or not the doctor was negligent is to be decided on the basis of the circumstances existing at the time of the claim of negligence. A doctor is not liable for an error in judgement if he does what he decides is best after careful examination and if it is a judgement which a reasonable, prudent doctor could or would have made under the circumstances in this case."

What the hell was I listening to? The doctor doesn't have to be held to any specific standards, it's okay if he's an idiot as long as there are other doctors that are idiots? It's okay if he harms someone as long as he used the level of judgement that he was capable of, even if it was an error?

He is not responsible to make sure he gives the best of care, only reasonable care? If there is a bad result because of his poor judgement, oh well, he didn't have to give you a guarantee anyway? I wasn't concerned about these words for our case, because I knew we had proven Dr. Proper's negligence far beyond the requirements of the law. People are convicted on murder charges beyond a reasonable doubt with far less evidence than was presented to this jury. However it deeply concerned me that a victim of a doctor's negligence was made to start out on their bare knees, and climb a very steep up-hill battle, only to have words like these hit them in the face when they reached the top. Who designed these jury instructions, a panel of negligent doctors? How could our legal system support such nonsense? Did the legal and medical systems sleep together? This was shocking and a very rude awakening for me. These are the people you trust your life with, should they not be held to even higher standards than others?

The Judge continued, and amongst these instructions was the measure of evidence needed in this case. "This is not a criminal case, so the plaintiffs do not have to prove their position beyond a reasonable doubt. The standard of proof involved in this case is called by a preponderance of evidence. That is, if, from all the evidence, including any evidence introduced by the defendant, you conclude that it is more probable that the defendant was negligent and that such negligence was a substantial factor in bringing about the injury, your finding on this issue will be for the plaintiff. If, however, you do not conclude or you find that the evidence is so evenly balanced that you are unable to say that there is a preponderance of the evidence on either side, your verdict must be for the defendant." When the judge had concluded his instructions, the jury left the courtroom to begin deliberations. I went to the bathroom to vomit.

The first time we heard from the jury was at 3:15 p.m. They made a request for a list of the witnesses who had testified.

The jury was brought back into the courtroom, and the foreperson was asked to rise and give their identity. The jury foreman was Mr. James French. Suddenly, all of those uneasy feelings came rushing back. It seemed that I couldn't get past one dreadful feeling without running right smack into the face of another. The stress was incredible, and I truly didn't know, mentally or physically how much more I was capable of taking.

It was now just short of five o'clock, and the judge had the jurors brought back into the courtroom. He asked them if they wanted to continue deliberations or preferred to continue in the morning. Mr. French stated that they would continue Thursday morning. During this conversation, my attention was drawn to the actions of another juror, Mr. Joseph Capezzuto. Mr. Capezzuto was staring at me, and when I looked back at him, he immediately dropped his head towards the floor in front of him. Keeping his head down, he brought his eyes back up toward me. He was trying to tell me something, and I knew it wasn't good. Since the beginning of the trial, from the very first witness on, I knew that the evidence was overwhelming on our behalf. Certainly this jury couldn't have had any doubt as to what had happened. But Mr. Capezzuto's actions had now left me very confused. I suddenly felt forced to entertain the thought that things may not go our way. I also knew my son Joe had been struggling to control his anger during the entire trial, and I was concerned about his reaction if the verdict was not in our favor. I approached John Falk, who, although was second chair to Angelo had been sitting in the audience of the courtroom during the trial. I expressed my concerns to John, and asked him if he would be sure to sit next to Joe when the verdict was read. John agreed to stay near him should he need to be physically restrained.

Court was dismissed until morning, and I went home. It was an absolutely horrible evening, and an even worse night. I couldn't eat or sleep, and my concentration was completely impaired. My mind kept jumping from one thought to another. I felt so weak and so desperate for rest, yet I couldn't stop thinking. The thought of Mr. Capazzuto kept running through my mind over and over again. What was he trying to tell me? What was going on in that jury room? Could there really be a chance that Dr. Proper could walk away from what he had done? With all the evidence presented to this jury, it would take a complete idiot not to see the truth. Could it be possible for six of them to have ended up on the same jury?

I finally dozed off to sleep, and immediately fell into a nightmare. In my dream I was walking down the stairs into the cellar of my home, and suddenly the walls started to swell like large marshmallows closing in on me. I was already trapped as I felt the walls squeezing my body, and I struggled to reach a window leading to the outside. I quickly punched a hole in it, pressing my face to the hole so I could breathe. As I felt the pressure of the walls on my body, I was gasping for air, and could barely whisper for help. I suddenly woke up sobbing, and my body was now shaking uncontrollably. I thought, Dear God, please don't let me face the pain of watching him get away with what he's done.

The next morning the jury continued deliberations. They requested to hear Linda Moore's testimony from the time of the extubation to the time that CPR began, and also the definition of Negligence and Preponderance of evidence. They were given both pieces of information, but it wasn't clear what they were focused on. Linda Moore had testified that she didn't see Dr. Proper actually extubate Joe, and only realized there was a problem when she saw Dr. Proper trying to force air into Joe's lungs with the mask. As for the definition of negligence, Dr. Proper could have strangled him in front of her, and if he felt it was the right thing to do at the time, and according to the definition, it was acceptable. The preponderance of evidence meant, "More likely than not." Once again, we would sit and wait.

At 2:10 p.m. we were called back into the courtroom. This time the jury had a verdict.

The clerk asked the foreperson to rise, and Mr. French stood up. She then read the charge. "In the matter of Joseph V. Nucci, by his Guardian, Linda Nucci, and Linda Nucci, individually, as plaintiffs, against Gilbert Proper, M.D., and the Rochester General Hospital, as defendants, have you reached a verdict?" Mr. French: "Yes, we have."

Then the Judge spoke, "In answer to question number one: Was the defendant, Dr. Gilbert Proper, negligent, what is your verdict?" Mr. French: "NO."

There was a low roar of gasps throughout the courtroom. Stunned was a gross understatement to describe everyone present. The Judge sat at the bench with his mouth literally hung open. I could hear Angelo next to me repeating over and over "I'm so sorry, I'm so sorry." I couldn't move. I just sat, as though frozen in time, as I looked at all the jurors. Mr. James French, a bakery manager at Wegmans. Mr. Robert Cole, a contractor at John Betlem Heating and Cooling. Debbie Newman, a lab technician at South Towne Veterinary Hospital, Robert Carr, a contractor at Brown's Race Insulation Service, Daniel Juers, an employee at Dupont, and Joe Capezzuto, a coordinator with the Rochester City School District. Their names, faces, and stupidity would be imbedded in my mind forever.

Although it felt like an eternity, the silence was finally broken by the screams of my son Joe. He stood up facing the jury and screamed "Are you kidding me, are you fucking kidding me!" and then, as I had suspected, he started to lunge towards Dr. Proper screaming "I'll kill him, you won't get away with this you fucking bastard, I'll kill you!" Mr. Falk and several others grabbed him and took him out of the courtroom. Now I was shaking inside and out, and although I didn't want Joe to openly display such anger, I had to admit I was feeling the same way. I walked over to Dr. Proper and stood directly in front of him. I leaned forward and said "I hope you see my husbands face in your sleep every night for the rest of your life, because you know exactly what you did." Dr. Proper kept his head down, and his eyes fixed on the table below him. He would not look up at me, and Mr. Brown did the same, holding his hand over his brow. I could hear Angelo saying,

"Lin, No." I said, "He knows exactly what he did, and he's just a lying bastard."

As we left the courtroom the reality was starting to kick in for everyone. My daughter Daneane was crying so hard she was hyperventilating. I felt like I was in slow motion as I watched several people trying to help her to catch her breath. Once I saw that she was okay, I realized I couldn't find my son Joe. He was nowhere in sight. "Where is Joe, I asked," and Nick, who was next to me said, "Mom, he's not here, let him be alone right now." As we stood there, a young lawyer from the District Attorney's Office, who had been following the trial, came up to me and said, "I've lost murder cases that haven't made me feel like this, I feel like I just took a bullet in my heart." Another Supreme Court Judge, who was also present in the courtroom throughout the trial and during the verdict, came up to me to express his disbelief.

I said, "How could they let him walk away with this, how could they not see he was lying?" and the Judge responded, "The whole damn courthouse knew he was lying, I don't know what was wrong with this jury." Angelo then walked up to us and said, "Well Judge, we did our best, but he did it again, he raped her again." He couldn't have used a more appropriate choice of words. That's exactly how I felt, like I had been brutally raped, and then publicly raped again when seeking justice. Feeling overwhelmed, I began walking through the courthouse aimlessly. My son Nick followed me, and then he just held me while I cried. He said, "Don't cry Mom, we've gotten through so much in life, we'll get through this too." As he was trying to console me, I could see he was crying as well. My poor son, his heart was broken, yet through his own pain, he was trying to hold me together. Knowing what a beautiful person he is made me hurt even more.

CHAPTER XV

The following Thursday Angelo appeared before Judge Syracuse to appeal the verdict. I couldn't bear the thought of stepping back into a courtroom. I harbored very bitter feelings for this thing called " Justice," and I refused to attend. Thoughts of the trial just wouldn't leave me, and I had exhausted myself, spending every minute of every day searching for the answer that could have brought the jury to this conclusion. I thought that if I could understand and justify why they had chosen not to find him responsible, it would help me to accept their verdict, and that acceptance might in turn put me on a path to healing. I needed to objectively review each piece of evidence presented to them, and to acknowledge that my personal pain and anger may have blinded me from seeing other views. I knew this wouldn't be easy, but I was desperate and determined to find something that could give me some peace of mind.

As I reviewed the testimony of each witness, I kept my focus on looking for facts that could suggest Dr. Proper's innocence. I put the witnesses in the order they had appeared in court, and made a list of their key statements. As hard as I truly searched, this wasn't working. I couldn't find one piece of evidence to support Dr. Proper's theory, and that included the statements of the defense experts, whose theories Angelo had clearly destroyed on the witness stand. There was just no feasible way six people could have honestly made this decision, unless they collectively shared one feeble brain. I now had stronger feelings than ever that something very sinister had taken place involving this jury. I couldn't stop thinking how Mr. Brown's attitude had been so inappropriate. He knew damn well the testimony proved his client's guilt, could it be he was not concerned because there was an alternate plan in place? I thought about the bathroom encounter. Why had Mr. Brown and Dr. Proper been in there with Mr. French, and why were they smiling as they came out? Was the fact that Mr. French refused to look at Nick during his testimony some kind of a signal to them? What really went on during that six-day delay? To make the matter worse, when the trial was over, one of the jurors had been interviewed about the verdict. The juror told the lawyer that when they arrived in the jury room to begin deliberations they took an initial vote. The vote was four to two that Dr. Proper was guilty. Two of the jurors argued very strongly on behalf of the defense. Those two jurors, were Robert Carr, and of course, James French. These two men had spent the entire deliberations convincing the other four jurors that Dr. Proper was innocent. The other jurors finally conceded to their opinions. Could Dr. Proper really be the luckiest person on the face of this earth? Could the only two people in the world lacking the ability to see the truth really have ended up together on the same jury? What was the reason they were so driven to convince the other jurors that he was not responsible? I had watched this unfolding all along before my own eyes, and I knew without a doubt that there were more serious issues involved than just this verdict.

It was now Friday morning, the day after the appeals. At approximately 9:30 a.m., I received a phone call from Mr. Faraci's secretary, Ann. Ann informed me that Judge Syracuse had set the verdict aside. I asked her what that meant, and she stated that the Judge had ruled for no verdict, and the case should be retried. All I could say was "Thank you God, thank you for allowing this Judge to see the truth, thank you for giving him the integrity to do something about it." His ruling, of course, would be subject to appeals in higher courts by the defense, but I was glad that the hospital, the lawyers, and Dr. Proper knew it wasn't over. The truth was so obvious it would take more than playing with the jury to just walk away from this one. However, as I thought about the Judges ruling, I developed a feeling of bitter sweet. I couldn't accept the thought of Dr. Proper not being held responsible, yet the thought of going through another trial terrified me. Once again, I was on another emotional roller coaster. The one thing I knew for sure, should there be another trial, I would voice my concerns, and make a request to have the next jury sequestered.

I met again with Mr. Faraci to get the details of what was going to happen next. He explained that the appeals process could be a very long ordeal. We were probably looking at another year or more before we would be back in court again. He also informed me that he had filed appeals to Judge Syracuse on both the weight of the evidence, and on the fact that Kathy Bellucco's testimony was eliminated because of the "Hearsay ruling" Judge Syracuse had made during the trial. Judge Syracuse chose to set the verdict aside on the basis of his erroneous ruling not to allow Kathy to testify. He claimed that his ruling was incorrect, and that the jury needed to hear her testimony. In his Memorandum Decision filed with the Appellate Court Judges, he stated the following: "Since a new trial is required it is unnecessary for the Court to consider the plaintiffs' arguments regarding the weight of the evidence."

Angelo told me he had hoped that the ruling would have been made on the weight of the evidence because the courts in New York are very conservative on issues of hearsay. I knew he was gently trying to tell me that we were once again facing another up-hill battle.

Judge Syracuse was a very respected judge amongst his peers, and carried a reputation for fairness, and for rarely rejecting a jury's verdict. I'm sure he was well aware of the conservative views of the Appeals Courts in New York regarding hearsay issues. He must have felt very strongly that his ruling of Kathy, as a hearsay witness was not only incorrect, but that her testimony clearly did not fall within the usual constraints of the hearsay laws. Kathy not only had valuable information to offer, but the fact that all the parties were present in court and that she would have been subject to cross-examination, eliminated the usual threats posed by a hearsay witness. One could also speculate that Judge Syracuse might have believed if he admitted an error on his part, and had given more than good cause to reverse this error, his reputation would also lend weight to the decision of his peers, and they would in turn support his ruling. At the very least, they should respect the fact that it was he who had presided over this trial and had listened to the testimony of all the witnesses. Who could be better qualified to determine if the case should be retried.

CHAPTER XVI

Angelo got busy working on the appeal, and I got busy filing a complaint with the New York State Dept. of Health Professional Medical Conduct Board. Angelo thought I was crazy to do this after four years had passed, but, there are no statute of limitations on filing a complaint, and I had good reasons for doing this now. When a doctor is found guilty of malpractice in a court of law, this board automatically investigates the doctor's conduct. With the verdict this jury had now rendered, I needed to file a formal complaint in order to have his conduct investigated. I would do everything I could to have him stripped of his license. I didn't want him ever to have the opportunity to harm another person, and I wasn't willing to wait to complete another trial for that to happen. I had already wasted enough time waiting for the completion of the first trial, confident that any jury could see the truth.

I obtained the necessary forms, and filled them in with the following complaints:

1. Dr. Proper exercised poor medical judgement by prematurely extubating Joe after his surgery, thus causing laryngospasms to occur.

2. Dr. Proper failed to provide Joe with continuous monitoring post operatively, both physically as well as with mechanical apparatus,

thereby allowing Joe to suffer an undetected lengthy time of anoxia, resulting in severe and permanent brain damage.

3. Dr.Proper failed to transfer Joe to a safe area post operatively within an acceptable time frame and failed to provide measures to insure his safety during the delay.

4. Dr. Proper allowed a room turnover to proceed with Joe still in the operating room, thereby engaging in a deviation from accepted medical practice.

5. Dr. Proper failed to call a code or summon help although aware that help was very badly needed.

6. Dr. Proper lacked the ability to properly manage Joe's airway, and provide him with oxygen in a timely manner consistent with life.

7. Dr. Proper refused to communicate, verbally or via documentation, any facts surrounding the stated event, and engaged in the altering of medical records.

Included with the form the DOH had sent me for the Professional Medical Conduct Board, was a separate form, to which I could list complaints against the hospital as well. This form would be forwarded to the Hospital and Primary Care Program of the Dept. of Health. I knew that if the hospital had filed an honest report with the DOH at the time of the incident, as they are required to, they would have been forced to take disciplinary action on Dr. Proper. I also realized that if the hospital did enforce any disciplinary actions on him, they would be admitting his guilt. The hospital had loyalty to no one, but the smarter choice here, was to ignore Dr. Proper's conduct, support his claim of innocence, and attempt to alter or delete any information that could prove otherwise. This choice would better serve to strengthen the hospitals position for the lawsuit they knew was coming, and this was far more important to them than what Dr. Proper had done.

I listed several complaints regarding the hospitals conduct. Aside from the covering up of Dr. Proper's conduct, I stated that Joe's medical records had been altered, a room turnover had progressed with Joe still in the operating room, and that the hospital was aware of both and had not taken issue with either.

When I filed these accusations against the hospital, my hope was to direct the attention of the DOH to the section of Joe's chart that contained the many time changes and how boldly they were written over. I knew it was unacceptable to alter a medical document in the manner in which they had done. I was also hoping they would find the lack of documentation of the event, including the incomplete code sheet unacceptable. I knew the chart wouldn't contain documentation that would offer any proof of the room turnover that had taken place, but if concerned enough, they may take the initiative to dig a little deeper than just the charting.

These were legal documentation issues that fell within the scope of the Dept. of Health's authority. I also knew that the DOH investigator would need the section of Joe's chart at the time of his surgery in order to complete an investigation of these complaints. If this section was missing it would send up a red flag to the investigator, and the hospital would be forced to produce it, or explain why it wasn't there, which could create another issue for the DOH to address with them. Aware that the hospital didn't play by any rules, I didn't want to leave them with the ability to remove this information from the chart. Being a nurse, I knew what the rules were, and if the hospital could do this to me, I shuddered to think what they were capable of doing to others. I wondered how many times information had been altered or disappeared if it wasn't to their advantage. How many people had they cheated from the truth?

I also knew that individually, each one of my allegations may not produce more than a slap on the wrist for the hospital, but collectively these allegations could paint a picture of deceit that may strike a concern in someone of authority at the DOH. Maybe that someone could, and would, be willing to take issue with that concern. Realistically, I knew that was a very big maybe. If nothing else, I wanted the hospital to feel the heat of an investigation by the Dept. of Health. I wanted to make it difficult for them to do this to anyone else. If enough complaints were filed against the hospital, eventually the DOH would be forced to take a serious look into their conduct.

Almost a year had passed before the Dept. of Health responded to my complaint. I received a letter that said due to legal issues, they were not able to share any of the details of their investigation with me, but after conducting a "Very Thorough" investigation into my allegations, they had concluded that Rochester General Hospital had done nothing wrong. I was disappointed with this response, but it was exactly what I had expected. What I didn't expect was that they concluded their letter by extending me their condolences on the "Death of my husband." I was absolutely outraged! The very organization in place to police the hospital's conduct had about as much credibility as the hospital itself. Now I certainly didn't hold much hope for the Professional Medical Conduct Board with their investigation of Dr. Proper. I knew they were just a different division of the same organization.

Almost another year had passed when an investigator from the Professional Medical Conduct Board called to inform me that my case against Dr. Proper was being reviewed. She explained that there were only a handful of investigators, and told me how overwhelmed they were with many cases. She said she had no idea how long it would be before my case would be completed. She also informed me that if they didn't find enough evidence to suspend or revoke Dr. Proper's license, it was within their discretion to take other disciplinary action on him that neither the public nor I would ever be privy to. She also said I shouldn't be discouraged if I didn't get the result that I was looking for, because it was their experience that where there's smoke there was usually fire, and more than one complaint would reopen previous cases. I was already discouraged by what she had told me. I informed her that the purpose of this investigation was to stop Dr. Proper from harming someone else, not to wait until he did, so they could file a complaint as well. Why should he be given even one more opportunity to destroy another life? I also informed her about the response I had received from the DOH regarding their supposed "Thorough investigation" of the hospital, and how I was hoping that her organization would be more credible.

CHAPTER XVII

January 25th 2000, Angelo appeared before the Appellate Judges to present his arguments to uphold Judge Syracuse's ruling for a new trial. This time I did attend. Although Angelo was limited to addressing only the fact that the jury should have been allowed to hear the testimony of Kathy Bellucco, he did manage to bring up some of the very strong evidence suggestive of guilt that had been presented during the trial. He argued that the exclusion of Kathy's testimony had not only prevented the jury from the benefit of hearing the information she had to offer, but had also prevented his cross-examinations of both Tammy Higgins and Debbie Fader. This ruling had prevented him from eliciting valuable information from them that the jury should have heard before deciding their verdict. Angelo further argued that Kathy's testimony was an exception to any of the existing hearsay laws, because all of the parties involved were present in court, and the defense had the ability to cross-examine her and dispute any information she had to offer. The jury should have been allowed to hear her testimony and determine what they believed to be the truth. He stated that Judge Syracuse recognized that he had made an error in his ruling of her as a "hearsay witness," and because of this error he had now ordered a new trial. Angelo reminded them that Judge Syracuse had listened to all the evidence at the trial, and it was he who was in the best position to determine if he had erred. Angelo strongly urged them to uphold his decision. For the most part, his argument contained the same information that Judge Syracuse had forwarded to these Judges in his memorandum. Angelo also cited previous cases that had already been ruled as exceptions to the hearsay laws for various reasons, the presence of all the parties in the court, and the ability to cross-examine being one of them.

Of course the defense argued that in spite of the absence of Kathy's testimony, the jury had heard all of the evidence they needed to hear during the trial, and had made their decision based on that evidence. I wondered what gave the defense the authority to determine how much evidence was needed. They asked that the original ruling of Kathy as a "Hearsay witness" be upheld. They requested that these Judges overturn Judge Syracuse's order for a new trial, and honor the jury's verdict of not responsible.

The Appellate Judges needed only to base their decision on the issue of hearsay, and not address the issues of the evidence. If they chose to opine that Kathy was a hearsay witness, then the jury's verdict would be upheld. If they chose to opine that Kathy's testimony was in fact an exception to the existing hearsay laws, then we would get the opportunity for a new trial.

At the completion of the arguments, Angelo expressed to me that he was hopeful. Not only did Kathy's testimony clearly fall within the exceptions of the hearsay laws, but that the defense had failed to present any arguments on the basis of any previous hearsay rulings.

Angelo then told me that it could be six to eight weeks before we would have this courts ruling, and win or lose, we may still be facing yet a higher Court of Appeals. The next Court of Appeals was the last step in the legal process, and you could only appear before them if they granted permission to hear your arguments.

This was all getting very complex for me. It wasn't even clear to me why this hearsay ruling was allowed to become an issue in the first place. If Kathy was considered a hearsay witness, then aside from the experts, so were many of the other witness who had testified. Wasn't it obvious there was a reason the defense had argued so vigorously to prevent just her testimony from being heard? Even knowing they had the opportunity to cross-examine her, they didn't want the jury to hear what she had to say. I could only hope that these Judges were the fair and intelligent people they were expected to be.

Four weeks later, we received their decision. They decided that Kathy was in fact a hearsay witness, and rejected Judge Syracuse's order for a new trial. So much for fair and intelligent, but as disappointed as I was, I couldn't help but think how Judge Syracuse felt. These Judges had spit disrespect in his face, and he made it known that he was furious about it. I wondered if he now realized that the weight of the evidence did need to be addressed, as Mr. Faraci had requested. Although obvious that Kathy should not have been considered a hearsay witness, if the evidence could have been argued, Angelo would have had a mountain of issues to work with. Now he was confined to one legal issue, with the evidence not needing to be considered at all.

A short time later the Court of Appeals granted Angelo permission to hear our case.

CHAPTER XVIII

Once again Mr. Faraci started preparing yet another appeal. This time he did provide a very detailed explanation of the incident for the Judges, with hopes that they would acknowledge the facts of the case. He explained that Joe's surgery was approximately one hour longer than expected, and the operating room he was in was needed for an emergency surgery. This was the reason Joe had been transferred from the OR bed to the floor bed, quickly extubated, and was then left without oxygen, unmonitored, and unattended, while the staff hurried to prepare for the next surgery. As the staff busied themselves, documenting, removing used instruments, and getting organized for the next case, Joe was left on the floor bed in another area of the room, out of their way. A room turnover was then called, with Joe still in the room. Anesthesia technicians Tammy Higgins, and Debra Fader responded to that call, and while in the room, both had observed Joe to be blue before any resuscitative efforts had begun.

It was Debra who spoke up and said, "Is this suppose to be this way? Is something wrong here?" It was only then that the doctors and nurses turned around and rushed to start putting the breathing tube back in him, and that's when "All the ruckus broke out." Tammy had verbalized this information to Kathy, and others, just two days after the incident took place, and before the defense had the opportunity to suppress her statements. Kathy's direct testimony would have opened the door for Angelo to cross-examine both Debra and Tammy on these statements, and allow the jury to hear this information as well. This was not only compelling, but was also the only direct evidence we had to prove that Dr. Proper had breached his duty to continuously monitor Joe by direct observation and with instruments, and to maintain his airway. The only other direct testimony about what Dr. Proper was doing during this crucial period came from Dr. Proper himself, as others present in the OR at that time, had displayed an incredible lack of memory during the trial. Furthermore, Dr. Proper's actions immediately after the crisis were inconsistent with the defense he asserted at trial. Dr. Proper had told a different story to the surgeon, the attending physician, and to the family regarding the amount of time Joe was without oxygen. His defense at trial was that Joe's obstruction was quickly turned around, but that he suffered brain damage from an unrelated EMD, which prevented oxygen from reaching his brain for 9 to 15 minutes. This testimony was contrary to the testimony and the results of the tests performed by the hospital Cardiologist, and that EMD was never diagnosed as the cause of Joe's condition outside of the litigation process. During trial, Dr. Proper also testified that "I did realize that Mr. Nucci had anoxic brain damage," yet failed to communicate that to Dr. Wojdylo right after the crisis ended. In fact, Dr. Proper had informed Dr. Wojdylo that the crisis period was very brief, and never made mention of any incident of EMD. Mr. Faraci also included that all of the records, which were controlled by the defense, were unreliable, as they contained many changes in the times and sequences of events during the time of the crisis.

Reading Mr. Faraci's appeal once again made me feel hopeful. The facts of the case reeked with common sense, but I had become mindful that common sense was not something our judicial system indulged in. Common sense would have forced this jury to render a verdict of guilty. Common sense would have forced the Appellate Judges to see that Kathy offered valuable information that should have been heard by the jury and left open to cross-examination.

Once again, I hoped that the Judges in this Court of Appeals would acknowledge the facts that Angelo had provided to them. I found myself reflecting back on the story of Suzanna, and I hoped that these Judges had the same thirst for justice that King Daniel had, and that they too possessed the wisdom to see the distance between the trees. These were the people who had the ability to demand the truth, and put honesty back in the courtroom.

Mr. Faraci, once again expressed that he was hopeful. He told me, "If ever there was an exception to the hearsay rule it was this one, and if this one didn't prevail, the Judicial System in New York would probably never see another one that did." Again he reminded me that the courts of New York remained very conservative on hearsay issues. I should pray real hard, that the Judges would be open-minded enough to recognize the unfairness of the self-serving statements made by Dr. Proper.

CHAPTER XIX

July 27th 2000, I received my answer from the Professional Medical Conduct Board. The letter read as follows; "The Office of Professional Medical Conduct operates under the provisions of and within the constraints of the New York State Public Health Law, which requires that physicians meet "minimally" accepted standards of care. A comprehensive and thorough investigation, which included numerous interviews of medical and nursing personnel who were involved in the operating room, and careful review of the medical record, we found that the care rendered by Dr. Proper fell within acceptable standards of practice. We fully understand the nature of your complaint and are most sympathetic with your distress. However without the evidence to support your allegations and without findings of substandard care, we cannot pursue charges of professional misconduct "As defined by the law." Therefore, the investigation has been discontinued and the case is now considered closed. A permanent confidential record of this investigation will be retained on file in our office. If new complaints are received that show evidence of a pattern, your case may be reconsidered. Thank you for bringing your concerns to our attention."

This time I didn't even hurt. This time all I felt was disgust. They based this decision on the interviews of the liars in the operating room? They could have interviewed me, and I would have told them what they were going to say. A comprehensive review of a chart that glared with time changes, and information contrary to the test results, as well as the documentation of the doctors who had completed these tests? I had even provided them with copies of the sworn statements of Tammy Higgins, and Debra Fader. They had the nerve to send me their sympathy! I had to let them know how I felt, and I responded with the following letter:

Dr. Novello,

I wish to thank you for time spent in the investigation of Dr. Proper's conduct concerning my husband Joseph Nucci's care. However, if you are not capable of using your own medical expertise and professional knowledge to conclude what happened in the operating room after my husband's surgery was completed, then quite frankly you should be examining the purpose for the existence of your organization, as well as the value of your individual roles.

Records lie and people lie, and I was mistaken to believe that I could rely on your medical knowledge and integrity to sort through these lies and distinguish what very obviously did happen. This is one case where the outcome of the patient clearly dictates the chain of events that took place in the OR, and if you were thorough in your review of Joe's chart, the order of the events would have been be very obvious to you. Perhaps you were looking for the confession that wasn't documented.

Your keeping of a confidential record is of no consolation to me. This is like telling a murder victim's family that one murder doesn't count, so there can be no prosecution until the murderer establishes a pattern.

When a man can undergo abdominal surgery without complication and ends up in bradycardia secondary to hypoxia, as the events prove, and suffers the degree of permanent brain damage that Joe has, one must question what standards of care were practiced. Your decision tells me that it is acceptable for a doctor to extubate a patient too soon, and leave a patient unmonitored directly postoperatively and to leave him physically unattended. It is acceptable for a doctor not to be capable of reestablishing an airway in an acceptable time frame, in an operating room with everything he needs at hand. It is also acceptable for a room turnover to proceed in the OR with a patient still in the room, and acceptable to alter records to fit the time frame one designs after the fact.

The message your decision sends is, there are no standards of care, minimal or otherwise, and once again a cover up goes on, and the medical code of silence prevails, because even your organization isn't credible enough to break it.

The only question posed in this matter should have been was Dr. Proper negligent or was he incompetent, but I guess we'll have to wait for him to establish a pattern to find out.

I signed the letter on behalf of my husband.

This felt like one more kick in the face, and this time I knew it was coming. I was sad and frightened to find that this organization did not function in the best interest of the public. I hadn't filed empty accusations, these were facts, and anyone with the ability to read a medical chart could have recognized that Dr. Proper's claim of EMD was a far cry from the facts that the Cardiologist had now clearly documented. What did it take to make one man's life count? What gave them the right to give a doctor a second chance to destroy another life? Then it occurred to me that the Dept. of Health is an organization of doctors. Of course they're reluctant to take down one of their own. They would bend every rule possible to protect their fellow doctors, and ultimately they were protecting themselves as well. And now I knew where the Judge's jury instructions came from. The New York State Public Health Law should be called The New York State Doctors Health Law. Who protects the public if doctors are the only ones they're interested in serving?

CHAPTER XX

It was another year before Mr. Faraci was scheduled to present arguments in the Court of Appeals. I was fighting a constant emotional battle, and I wanted it to end. From the moment this tragedy happened I had never spent one day of my life feeling sorry for myself. Tragic things happen to good people everyday, and life certainly offered no guarantee that I would be excluded from that. I accepted that, but I wasn't willing to accept the lack of accountability. I wasn't willing to accept the lies, and I knew I would never forgive either. Feelings of anger wouldn't leave me, and hate was growing inside me like a cancerous tumor that only the truth could destroy. I now hated the jurors as much as I hated Gilbert Proper. I hated some for their ignorance and stupidity. I hated others for their lack of morals. I hated all of them for turning their backs on what they knew was the truth, and I hated them for this road to hell that I was made to travel because of their incompetence. Had they been competent, all of this could have ended right in that courtroom. I carried a constant knot in the pit of my stomach. I was getting bitter, and bitter hurts.

February 14th 2001, I was sitting on the couch in my living room, and my son Nick went outside to get the mail. He walked back into the house and stood in the foyer. He had an opened letter in his hand that he was reading. Speechless, he looked up from the letter and just stared at me with a painful look of disbelief on his face. I felt my stomach immediately rush to my throat. I couldn't move, and I couldn't cry. All I could say was, No, No, No!

The next morning, I picked up the letter from Angelo and started to read. " Dear Lin, You can't imagine how I hate to write this letter." I burst into uncontrollable tears, and I just couldn't bring myself to read it.

The following day I did finish reading the letter. The Appeals Court had decided to uphold the Appellate Courts decision to rule Kathy as a hearsay witness. According to their written decision, they were well aware of the evidence in the case, but chose to lend more weight to the fact that Kathy was Joe's cousin, than to the value of her testimony. They felt that because she was Joe's cousin, she might have had a strong motive to shade her testimony.

Who the hell were they to make an assumption on Kathy's credibility. Does the fact that you're someone's cousin make you a liar? Does the fact that you're a doctor make you not a liar? Didn't Dr. Proper have stronger motive to shade his testimony than Kathy could ever have?

Furthermore, they stated that the conversation between Kathy and Tammy had taken place at a Nucci family gathering, which couldn't have been farther from the truth. Kathy was at a gathering with her new husband's family and friends, some of whom had also heard the statements made by Tammy, and they didn't even know the Nucci family. In fact, they barely knew Kathy. They also stated, that Tammy Higgins was a young, inexperienced high school student with no medical training. I still don't know what that had to do with anything. They didn't have any medical training either, but I'll bet that they, like anyone else past the age of five could identify the color blue. They didn't offer any excuse for Debra Fader, who had also seen that Joe was dark blue, and she was a very experienced anesthesia technician. Their final statement read as follows: We recognize that several states have chosen to adopt the so-called "modern" view - - permitting the admission of prior, unsworn oral statements where the declarant is available and subject to cross-examination, however, we retain our adherence to the traditional approach. Opinion by Judge Wesley. Chief Judge Kaye and Judges Smith, Levine, Ciparick, Rosenblatt and Graffeo concur.

How could adherence to a traditional approach hold more value than truth and justice? They were given the facts of the case, and they had clearly misused those facts. They chose to focus on the "possibility" of Kathy's testimony being shaded, yet they had no problem accepting the fact that Dr, Proper had given nothing but shaded testimony. If this was the highest level of intelligence in our Judicial System, then God help us all.When the people who wear the black robes in this country chose to hide behind the comfort of a "Traditional approach," then clearly they lack the insight and initiative to do their job. They need to be excused, and step aside for people more deserving to wear those robes. People who really care about the truth, and are willing to work at making a difference in the fairness of our Judicial System, and not just upholding lazy traditional approaches.

I wrote a letter, and expressed my feelings about their decision. I'm sure, if they even bothered to read it, I was discounted as some angry lady who was just upset because she didn't get her way. Quite frankly, I didn't give a damn what they thought. I don't feel one ounce of respect for any one of them. I didn't want to give them the comfort of their decision being just another "case over" that they could clear from their docket, and never have to think about again. I wanted to them to know that there are real people that hurt, and count on their ability to rise above lies and deceit. I told them that adhering to traditional approaches was just an excuse that allowed them to be lazy and ignore the truth, and that this laziness was exactly what some attorneys counted on in their attempts to manipulate the system.

I asked that when faced again with the same or similar situation that they consider putting an end to the traditional approaches that only served as catalysts for liars, as other states had already taken the initiative to do.

If I sounded like an angry lady, so be it, but if any of my words could impact their thoughts when making another decision, then maybe justice would be better served for others.

A week after I received his letter, I called Angelo. I thought he was confident that the Appeals Court decision would be favorable to us, as he had already started preparing for our next trial.

Although he would never tell me this, someone else did. I was sure this decision was eating him from the inside out, just as it was myself. In fact, I knew he carried the disappointment of this trial in his heart from the moment the jury rendered their twisted verdict.

I told him that I didn't appreciate the Valentine message that he sent me, and that I had waited all day for the bouquet of dead flowers to arrive. He chuckled and said, "Well at least you don't hate me." How could I ever hate him? This was a man who had done everything he possibly could to bring this case to justice. I know as an attorney it was his obligation to do his best, and I know that initially that was his plan, as he would with any other case. But I felt that his heart had gotten tangled up in this one. He had given so much of himself, and I came to believe that he didn't just want the win, he wanted the truth, and he had put both his mind and his heart into that fight for the truth. He was warm and caring, but had tried his best not to let me see that side of him.

He was brilliant and confident, yet at times humble, and his integrity was beyond impressive. When he fought in court he was prepared for all the dishonest testimony that he knew he would face, yet he himself would never step outside the boundaries of honesty. I believed in him, and that belief carried me through many times during the trial when I felt I couldn't make it. He fought for the truth with the truth, and win, or lose he is, and will always be my hero. I knew he would struggle with this painful outcome for a very long time, possibly forever, just as I would. The case was over, and we both needed to heal, but there remains a very special place in my heart that belongs to only him, and will for the rest of my life.

CHAPTER XXI

Several months had passed, but the anger of the losses stayed with me every minute of every day. Each time I looked at Joe I would think about how much he loved life, how much he loved his family, and how much we loved him. Every time he cried, my heart would sicken with thoughts that he was in a place that was far worse than death. And each time I would think about Dr. Proper enjoying his life, his career, and his family, and his ability to walk away freed from the responsibility of what he had done. As I struggled through each day, I would think about each member of the jury, and I couldn't imagine how these people were able to live with themselves.

I had now become very angry with God. There wasn't a reason good enough that he had turned his back on us so many times, and I refused to pray. I lost faith in everything I once believed in. Even the medical system that I had once been so proud of now felt so dirty. I was in a very empty and bitter place, and I knew if I stayed there, it was sure to destroy me. Once again, in my desperation to heal, I turned to the thought that I might be wrong. This time I knew I wasn't capable of making that judgement. I needed to find someone with the ability to review the case, and give me a completely honest opinion, but it had to be someone that didn't know us and could have no personal interest in the outcome of our case. If that someone could tell me that there was even a small possibility that I was wrong, I would accept that and move on.

I made contact with an old acquaintance. This was a person I knew was well respected, and was capable of giving me a completely honest opinion. Still, I didn't feel comfortable with the fact that he knew Joe, and many years prior had shared a working relationship with him. If I were to accept another's opinion, it would have to be from a complete stranger. I asked this acquaintance if he knew of any such person he thought might be willing to read the trial transcripts, and give me an honest opinion. He said he knew of one person with judgement he would trust that might be willing to do this. Later that same evening, that person called me. I felt uncomfortable asking this of someone I didn't know, but I was desperate, and feeling uncomfortable was the least of my concerns. We spoke very briefly and I shared none of my personal thoughts with him. I made arrangements to have the depositions and the trial transcripts delivered to his office.

There was a tremendous amount of material to read, and I knew it would take him quite some time to get through it. It was several months before I finally received a phone call from him. His said, "Are you kidding me! How the hell did you not win this case? Are you sure this jury was even alive" He went on for several minutes expressing his disbelief and how he felt that something was very wrong.

In my effort to find comfort and acceptance, I had managed to put myself into an even deeper anger. Here was that jury issue right back in my face again. I was convinced more than ever that something very sinister had to have taken place. I guess the defense was right when they argued that Kathy's testimony didn't matter, in fact now I'd bet my life that nobody's did.

As the months passed, I was busy making the necessary adjustments that I needed to in my life. I was terrified that I might be forced to put Joe in a Nursing Home, and that was something I knew I could never live with. He needed suctioned every fifteen to thirty minutes, and repositioned at a minimum of once an hour, for comfort and to prevent his skin from breaking down. We exercised him and put him in his wheelchair every day to stop him from becoming contracted. With constant observation we were able to quickly detect the onset of any pending illness and treat him quickly before he needed hospitalized. He has never spent one day in the hospital since the day he was discharged from St. Mary's. I knew there wasn't a medical facility in the world that could provide him with the constant care he needed. This is what his life had been reduced to. He had suffered enough, and he didn't deserve anything less than the best comfort I could possibly give him. With Dr. Grunspan's help I was able to obtain more hours of nursing service to care for Joe. I now had enough hours to allow me to work and to sleep, and I could take care of him myself in the remaining hours of the day. I was very grateful that this was possible, and that I was able to keep him at home. I also hoped that when the day of his passing finally came, I would be able to find some comfort in knowing that I had done everything I could to make his last years of life as comfortable as possible.

However, I wasn't grateful that Joe was now dependent on the state, with Medicaid being our only option to pay for his care. The Judicial System had relieved Dr. Proper and the hospital of their responsibility, and had placed the burden of his care on the people of the state. I took serious issue with the fact that the public was made to pay for something they had nothing to do with. This was especially difficult for me because of my new awareness that this was the public that no one chose to protect, but they were quick to dump the responsibility of a failed Medical and Judicial system on them.

Still bitter, I continued my struggle to put everything I had been through behind me. I tried all the different theories of healing that any good psychiatrist would recommend. I thought if I talked about it I would feel better, but talking about it only made me furious. Then I listened to the religious theory; "You can't heal if there is hate in your heart. You need to forgive." Well, where should I start forgiving? Should I forgive Dr. Proper for allowing my husband to suffocate until his brain was destroyed? Should I forgive him for all the pain and suffering his negligence has caused my family and myself? Should I forgive the fact that he's a lying coward? Should I forgive the others in the operating room who had also neglected Joe, and lacked the integrity and honesty to tell what really happened? Maybe I should forgive Mr. Brown, Mr. French, and Mr.

Carr, for what I will always know took place between them. I shouldn't forget to forgive the other jurors for being too gutless to hold their ground when they knew very well what the truth was. I could always forgive the Judicial System for not giving a damn about the truth, but they're still too busy trying to figure out who's qualified to identify the color blue, and they're far too lazy to care about justice. And maybe the DOH should be forgiven for not considering one man's life valuable enough to do anything about. They're waiting for more victims, so they can see a pattern. Forgiving was not something I was capable of doing.

Often people would ask me what went wrong, and I would simply answer, "You wouldn't believe me if I told you." Why would anyone believe me? I had lived through each one of these experiences, and I had a very hard time believing it myself. I would still on occasion question my own my ability to rationalize. I found it incredible that one person could experience as many disappointing outcomes as I had. In time I realized it was because I had reached out to so many in my plea for justice, and I wasn't prepared for any to reject the truth. I believed I was reaching to people who cared. I believed in the Judicial System, I believed it always supported the truth, and I never believed it would fail me. I believed in the DOH, and I believed it was created to protect all the people, not just doctors. I believed in people, and their ability to be honest and caring and to recognize the truth, and to act on that truth. The truth was that unless something affects someone personally, they really don't care. The sad reality is that at some point in life, not caring is certain to affect them personally.

I had learned many lessons in life, and had taken many hard blows in a short period of time, and it hurt like hell. I would often reflect on the words of someone who had once helped me through a difficult situation. A number of years ago, when faced with a small crisis in my life, I asked for the advice of someone I knew to be very wise. He said, "Be patient, life has a way of evening itself out," I was, and it did, and I know it will again.

CHAPTER XXII

Now I was left with only boxes of trial transcripts, and my shattered beliefs. For several months I kept those boxes of transcripts sitting on the floor in the family room of my home. Every day as I walked past them I would think to myself, "You need to put them away, out of sight." I knew that looking at them daily wasn't helping me to heal, but each day I would tell myself, " I'll put them away tomorrow."

One day I finally picked up the boxes and started to put them into storage. As I was putting them away, I realized that looking at them wasn't helping me, but putting them away wasn't helping anyone. I needed to share the facts of what happened with as many people as I could, and if knowing these facts could help even one person, it will have been worth my effort, and I started to write this book.

It was a Sunday morning in December 2002. When I awoke, I sat at the kitchen table with my cup of coffee, and I started to read the newspaper. I read that a young man in his early thirty's had undergone abdominal surgery at Rochester General Hospital, and was now in a coma. He had suffered an unknown duration of oxygen deprivation. The article stated that his family was looking for the answers to what had happened. I felt the coffee coming back up from my stomach, and I ran to the bathroom. Within minutes my phone started to ring with callers wanting to know if I had read the

article. One of these callers was my son Nick, and he was extremely upset. Nick had received a phone call from a friend who happened to be a close friend of the young man who had suffered this
tragedy. Nick's friend had spoken with the young mans father, who
had informed him that the hospital couldn't tell the family what had
happened, because they were having a difficult time locating the
information in his medical chart. Nick said, "Mom, when is someone going to stop them from getting away with this?"

What had started out as a search for personal justice now felt
like a crusade for the injustice I knew so many others have suffered,
and so many more were yet to suffer. Some may see the facts of this
story differently than I. Some may think I am irrational, or driven
by the pain of my experiences. Maybe some will think I am just an
angry lady who's not able to let go. But maybe God knew I would-
n't be able to let go, and maybe he never left my side after all,
because knowing I would share this information with you, may
have been his plan all along.

What others may think can't change my life, but I hope that
what I've told you may one day be able to save yours.

When a doctor stands before you, don't assume that his or her
title means they are capable of doing the right thing. Always
remember, they're not obligated to give you the best care, only
minimal care, and only they alone need to determine if that care is
sufficient. There are no "Standards of Care" to which they are made
to live up to, because the State will ignore all standards to protect a
doctor. Protocols are changed at will, and never on your behalf.

If a doctor makes an error in judgement and that error harms
you, or a loved one, you can be certain that the support of the New
York State Public Health Law is behind them, and not you. The
next time you read that a doctor's license has been revoked or sus-
pended, be certain to notice that it's only because he has a history
of repeated offenses. He has established the pattern the DOH
requires of him, and they have been forced to take action. Don't
allow yourself to become a victim of a pattern.

Get to know your doctor as a person, and if he doesn't allow
you the time to get to know him, that means he doesn't care to
know you. It's the doctor who sees you as a person and not just a

patient, who values your life. If you have the misfortune of being hospitalized, or have a sudden need for surgery, you may find yourself under the care of doctors you've never met before. Talk, ask questions, and let them know how you feel. Talking forces them recognize that you're a person, and not just another case they need to hurry and complete.

Don't accept care from a doctor who suddenly shows up and tells you what they're going to do, without offering you the opportunity or respect to answer your questions or listen to how you feel. He's in a hurry to get done, and don't accept that he's in a hurry to get done with you.

Tell your surgeon that you feel you are placing your life in their hands, and that you expect them to protect that life. Ask them to stay with you after your surgery until they are sure you are completely safe. If you make one doctor feel personally responsible for your life, they'll be less willing to rely on the judgement of others to protect you.

Use all of your instincts, and if something about the doctor doesn't feel comfortable to you, ask to see another one, it's your right. Ask them what they're going to do, ask why, and demand answers that you can understand. It's your life, don't be intimidated, chose your doctor, don't let them chose you.

If all your efforts to protect yourself or a loved one fails, and you end up in a court of law, don't believe that because you walk in with the truth, that the truth will prevail. Our Judicial System always perceives the doctor as the victim, and they take every measure possible to protect them, with little regard for your loss. The Judge will state that only the " Preponderance of evidence" is needed to determine if they have committed negligence, and will then deliver "Jury instructions" that almost guarantee they are relieved of all responsibility for their actions.

By no means is every doctor who stands accused of negligence guilty, but doctors, like every other profession, come with those that are good, those that are average, and those that just plain stink. While all are capable of making mistakes, all are not capable of telling the truth, and accepting responsibility for those mistakes. We need to let the State and the Courts know that we don't accept their support of lower standards that allow the ones that stink to hide behind the professionalism of the others.

If you should ever be called to serve on a jury in a medical malpractice case, welcome the opportunity. If the State is not willing to set higher standards to protect your life, or the lives of your loved ones, then use this opportunity to let them hear your voice. Let them know that you are not willing to accept ignored protocols and careless actions that put your lives as risk. Make your own laws. Let them know that you do expect the best of care, and are not willing to accept anything less.

Medical terminology can be very confusing and very intimidating, but common sense is not. When sitting on a jury, look past the attorneys attempts to confuse you. The more they use words like "Increased insurance rates" and "Frivolous lawsuits" the less truth they have to defend their clients with, and these comments have nothing to do with their client's guilt or innocence. They use these words, and others, as an attempt to further confuse you. Don't just hear what they say, hear what they don't say. If you still feel confused in your search for the truth, always look for the distance between the trees.